Dentists and Hov

Dentists and How to Survive Them

Barrie and Anne Sherman

Thorsons
An Imprint of HarperCollins*Publishers*

Thorsons
An Imprint of HarperCollins*Publishers*
77–85 Fulham Palace Road
Hammersmith, London W6 8JB

1160 Battery Street
San Francisco, California 94111–1213

Published by Thorsons 1996
1 3 5 7 9 10 8 6 4 2

Illustrations by Simon Batten

A catalogue record for this book
is available from the British Library

ISBN 0 7225 3216 4

Printed in Great Britain by
HarperCollinsManufacturing Glasgow

Contents

Acknowledgements

Few, if any, books have been written without the authors being in debt to the ideas and help of other people, and we are no exception to this rule. In alphabetical, rather than order of gratitude, we would like to thank Professor Bill Binnie, Mike Durcan, Alan French, Professor Stanley Gelbier, Richard Ibbotson, Philip Jepson, Claire Lincoln, Dr Eddie Lynch, Jane and Charlie Merrivale, Carl Nehammer, Professor Bernard Smith, an entirely unrelated Sue Smith and Geoff Taylor. Our indebtedness is the greater as their contributions to the book were invaluable. We would also like to thank Emma Waghorn for her meticulous editing. Last, but most definitely not least, we must thank Simon Batten for his fine illustrations, conceived and drawn from the perspective of the reader rather than the dentist. Any errors of omission or commission in this book are ours, not theirs.

Barrie and Anne Sherman, London 1995

Introduction

What do you really know about your mouth and teeth? Probably not as much as you should. And do you know what your dentist is actually doing when you lie back in that space-age chair? Almost certainly not, and you are not alone. This gap in your knowledge runs alongside a whole host of misconceptions and 'old-wives tales' about teeth and dentists.

This is surprising. After all, our mouths and teeth are in almost constant use, we see them every day, and for much of our lives we visit our dentist more often than our doctor. However, one thing is clear. You may not know much about them, but our mouths and teeth, and those of our children, are very important.

Teeth are crucial to the way we present ourselves to the world. When we meet someone the first thing we look at is the face, and at the least hint of a smile, the teeth. And we all respond well to smiles. Film directors have always known this. From the earliest days of cinema their heroes and heroines have had rows of even, shiny white teeth, but when the obvious heavies grin they show crooked teeth, gaps or broken, jagged stumps, and those with no teeth at all are cast as comedy characters.

When a photographer urges, 'Say cheese – smile', we know the photo will show exactly what our teeth look like. And have you ever noticed that in old portraits, royal families and other important people are never smiling? This is not only because they were supposed to look regal, it was also because if they smiled the painter would have had to show their rotting teeth, if they had any left at all. But nowadays this would be unthinkable. We expect to see all the people around us with 'Hollywood-style' rows of teeth, whether they are natural or have been manufactured in some way.

But teeth are not just a cosmetic convenience, like mascara or a toupee. The mouth is an important part of our bodies, which like the other parts needs to be kept in good order and healthy. It plays an important role in our general health. Despite the fact that modern processed foods are softer than ever before, we all need teeth to bite, tear and chew our food, if we are to have a balanced diet consisting of more than soup and yoghurt. If we are unable to eat efficiently our digestion suffers, and with it our general health and our ability to perform at our best. There are also times when small pockets of infection in the mouth not only result in pain and feelings of general ill health but also act as focuses for infection. And a healthy mouth is a sweet-smelling mouth, one without any of those embarrassing bad-breath odours that have people moving away from you as quickly, and as far, as they can.

Yet despite the fact that most people realize the overwhelming need to keep their mouths healthy, their breath fresh and their teeth and gums looking nice, few parts of the body are so taken for granted by their owners. It is just like a car. Once the newness has worn off, people tend to resent paying for a routine service when it is going well, only taking it to the garage when something goes wrong. And all too many people only notice their mouth and teeth when something goes wrong. But while a worn clutch can be replaced by a new one, with no difference in performance, teeth are not always so easily saved or repaired, and their replacements are never as good as the original models. It follows that keeping all your natural teeth 100 per cent intact is your 100 per cent best option.

This means not only that prevention is better than cure but also that regular dental checks, to ensure that any emerging problems are kept small, are the key to a healthy mouth and teeth. The problem is that the dental surgery comes well down the list of places that people choose to visit. Other than accidents and tooth fractures the most common way we know that all is not well in the mouth is pain, although bleeding gums, gumboils, the odd lump and comments about bad breath are also indications. This a bad start to a dental visit, especially if we believe that there may be even more misery to come. The mouth is a mysterious place. The level of pain that would have us saying, 'It's only a sprained ankle,' as we hobble away bravely, is excruciating when transferred to the mouth, while small spots on the cheek take on the proportions of the Alps, and it is impossible to stop the tongue from exploring them constantly.

The purpose of this book is to demystify the mouth, teeth and visits to the dentist. It aims to make you better informed both about your own teeth and about those of your children or other dependents, so that they can be kept as healthy and intact as possible. If this is no longer a possibility, the book explains the restorative and replacement alternatives, and the new methods of treatment and pain prevention now available in modern dental surgeries. This is an area where great technical and practical strides have been made over the past few years. By making more people aware of what is possible we hope this book will encourage people to go the dentist, and so save and repair their teeth.

The book is intended to be used for reference purposes by people with no prior knowledge of dental or mouth matters. It uses no jargon and explains those scientific and technical words and expressions we could not avoid using. Although we hope everyone will read the book from cover to cover, especially the sections on preventing dental disease, it is also designed to be kept handy and dipped into when the occasions arise, for example when a child's tooth has broken, at teething time, before a routine visit to the dentist, or when toothache strikes.

For easy reference the book is divided into three sections. The first is on the prevention of tooth and mouth disease. This will not only suggest self-examination but will also go through what a dentist looks for in his or her first check-up, and tell you how to find the dentist to do this initial examination. This is not always as easy as it sounds. Part One ends with a chapter on the sort of prevention that you can do for yourself, and help children to do, including diet dos and donts and the various ways of cleaning teeth, as well as how not to clean them.

Part Two is divided into age groups where different factors about teeth become important. This allows for easy and speedy reference whenever a problem or question arises. There is a chapter on babies and young children, one on young people, one on adults, and finally a chapter about the older mouth. Each chapter will deal with the sort of problems associated with each of these age groups.

Part Three is about what you may find at the typical

dentist. There are separate chapters on the people, the equipment, the sorts of materials, the different types of treatment you may come across, the future, and alternative dentistry. At the end of the book there is a glossary of technical words that you may have read in other places or may have overheard at the dentist.

All the indications are that the dental health of children in the UK is improving, and the younger the children the greater the improvement. Much of this has been attributed to the widening use of toothpastes with added fluoride. Yet not only are there 20 per cent of children whose teeth are actually getting more decay than ever, gum disease is now responsible for the majority of teeth lost in Britain.

There has also been a sea change in awareness of what can be done by dentists – in principle, if not in detail. For the first time, ordinary people are realizing that even very badly diseased teeth can be saved, rather than just extracted, and that fancy replacement work can now be done. In other words expectations for healthy mouths, and repaired or properly replaced teeth, have never been higher. This book is dedicated not only to maintaining those expectations but also to expanding people's dental horizons.

Part One

Prevention

Chapter One

The Personal Check-up

Self-examination is natural. Most of us do it every day. We check our faces in the mirror in the mornings and evenings (sometimes in-between), looking for wrinkles, blemishes and spots; and we check our hair for loss, greying, dandruff or split ends. Some of us note the colour of our tongues or the whites of our eyes at the same time. We check our hands for cuts or broken nails, and in the bath or shower check other parts of the body, such as breasts. But most of these are easy to see and, for the most part, we know what we are looking or feeling for.

We also clean our teeth at least once a day, or should do, and this is the perfect time to indulge in a spot of self-examination of the mouth and teeth. However, it has to be made clear at the outset that we wish neither to turn people into dental hypochondriacs nor to lead them to believe that their own efforts can replace those of dentists. The problem with self-examination is that few of us know exactly what we are looking for, and if we see nothing wrong we tend to believe that everything is all right. Unfortunately, as we shall explain, this may not be the case at all. It is important not to be lulled into a false sense of security. However, if we guard against complacency, we can use self-examination as a valuable way of spotting early signs of dental and mouth disease.

What to Look For

Colour Change

The first thing we can note is any change in the colour of our teeth. While it is easy to see whether this has happened to the front teeth, a strong light source is needed to see anything meaningful in the back of the mouth. You can buy an angled mirror rather like the one that dentists use, and with practice this may help. Colour changes can happen for several reasons. Heavy smokers know only too well that their teeth get stained. Some foodstuffs, red wine, turmeric, betel nuts and even tea also can discolour teeth severely; in fact, any food or drink that contains colouring can stain the *plaque* that coats uncleaned teeth. Some people may be taking medication that stains their teeth, but they should have been warned in advance that this might happen.

Plaque

These changes, however, are not the main focus of our interest. The most common sight is a whitish film, most easily seen on the front surfaces of the front teeth. You can scrape it off with a fingernail. This is not food debris. It is plaque. Like rust in cars it serves no useful purpose. We do not want it. It is the cause of both tooth decay and gum disease, so not unnaturally we shall come across it later in the book. Plaque is entering ordinary language – toothpastes and mouthwashes now advertise themselves as counteracting plaque. The main thing to say about it is that, if you see it, get rid of it by brushing it off. This, indeed, is the prime purpose of teeth cleaning.

Tooth Decay

Very badly decayed teeth are easy to see, and you will probably have felt pain from them before seeing them. Black holes and/or jagged edges make them difficult to miss. But at earlier stages some tooth decay (*dental caries*) stands out as a very white, roughish looking spot where the outer layer of the tooth (*enamel*) is starting to crumble. Later, decay can look like a dark shadow, or a dark spot or line on individual teeth. While these can be seen on the front surfaces of the front teeth, and between these teeth as well, they are far harder to see on the back ones.

This brings us to an important point. Each tooth has five surfaces, although the front eight teeth (the top and bottom *incisors*) have a fine edge as their fifth surface, and the teeth next to them (the four *canines*) are pointed. While you can easily see the front and biting surfaces of the back teeth you cannot see between them. Unfortunately this is where much of our tooth decay starts.

A major problem of decay is that although it might appear to be a very small patch on the outside of a tooth it may well have spread a great deal inside the tooth. In this way it is just like a rotten apple. The bug enters through a tiny break in the apple skin and creates a lot of destruction inside the apple before it gets big enough to show the extent of the damage on the outside. We only find that out after we have bitten into it. This is why you can have an apparently healthy tooth one day, but bite something hard and find the tooth has broken in half the following day.

We must emphasize that because you cannot see anything wrong, it does not mean that everything is all right. Finding colour changes tells you that something is wrong – finding no colour changes doesn't tell you that everything is well. If you can see things starting to go wrong get in touch with your dentist. And if things look all right to you, you should still go for your next regular dental check-up.

Tooth Structure

At this point it is useful to describe the structure of a tooth. Figure 1 (below) shows a cross section through a front tooth (a canine). There are two main parts of the tooth: the crown and the root. Front teeth have a single root; back teeth have two or three roots.

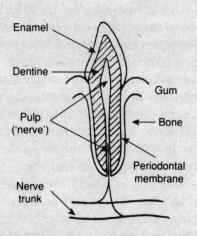

Figure 1 Cross section through a front canine

- The crown of a tooth is covered by a layer of *enamel*. It is the part of the tooth that you see. It is a hard substance made up of calcium and other mineral salts. It has no nerve supply so cannot transmit pain.
- Inside this, and inside the root, is the *dentine*. This is softer than enamel, can transmit pain and is where decay really spreads out.
- The root of the tooth is covered by another hard substance called *cementum*. Like enamel it is insensitive.
- The tooth is attached to the jaw bone by strong fibres that run into the cementum on one side and the outer layer of bone on the other. The whole suspension mechanism is called the *periodontal membrane*. Gum disease ultimately weakens these fibres.
- The *pulp* of the tooth runs down the centre of the tooth and carries the blood supply and nervous tissue. This is popularly known as the 'nerve'.

Dead teeth also change colour, often to an opalescent battleship grey. This is very noticeable in front teeth – and will drive most people to the dentist to see what can be done. It is important to realize that we are looking for *changes* to tooth colour. Some people have a natural mottling of white or yellowish colour on their teeth. We shall explain about this in Chapter 6, but for the moment the important fact is that this is not decay, nor does it necessarily weaken the teeth.

Calculus

You may see a greeny or greyish yellow deposit – sometimes a line – around the teeth next to the gum, especially on the inside of the front ones and the outside of the back teeth. It is hard and rough, and unlike plaque it is impossible to brush off. This is what used to be called tartar. It is now called *calculus*. We explain how it is formed in Chapter 8, page 73. It is similar in nature to limescale (fur) in a kettle or shower head. But it must be cleaned in a non-chemical way at your dentist. Never try to do it yourself. Calculus is a part of gum disease, which, as we observed in the introduction, is the most common cause of lost teeth.

Bleeding

Blood is another signal of things going wrong with the gums – blood on the toothbrush after teeth cleaning, blood on an apple or other hard food after biting, and perhaps blood on the pillow in the morning. It is a signal every bit as persuasive as toothache that a visit to the dentist is well overdue.

Checking Children's Teeth

All the above checks should always be made on behalf of children. It is also a good idea to get them to look for signs of trouble themselves from an early age. There is one additional check to be made on children. This involves the position of the teeth. It is worth looking for signs that the second teeth are set in crooked patterns or perhaps the upper or lower front teeth protrude excessively. This does not apply to milk teeth. While, as we shall see, straightening teeth (orthodontic treatment) generally starts from the onset of puberty, it is always wise to get to a dentist at the first signs of the problem, to enable professional monitoring, or treatment, as early as possible.

Other Mouth Problems

It is a common misconception that people with no teeth at all need not worry about the state of their mouth. Dentures can become ill-fitting over time, as the bones in the mouth change shape, causing ulcers or hard sore patches. Tooth roots buried for years can work themselves to the surface like fossils in a peat bog. And the same sorts of ulcers or small lumps and bumps in the mouth can occur whether you have all your teeth or no teeth.

Any painful or worrying lumps, ulcers, hard patches or discoloration (generally whitish) that stay around for more than two weeks, whether they are on the cheeks, gums or tongue, should send you to the dentist. The odds are greatly stacked against any of these being serious, but it is always better to be safe than sorry. Treat them with the respect you would give a mole that suddenly appears or expands. We shall deal with lumps and bumps in more detail in Chapter 8.

Other Signals

Self-examination goes beyond just looking. Clearly pain tells you that something is wrong, as does the presence of abscesses on the gums (also known as gumboils). These can be very painful. Teeth that become sensitive, especially to hot and cold or sweet things, are asking you to get something done, as is halitosis (bad breath). And a persistent nasty taste in the mouth may indicate gum disease or a long-lasting abscess that is draining into the mouth. We shall cover all of these in Chapters 7, 8 and 13.

There are also some diseases (chickenpox is an example) that have signs that show in the mouth, but this is a matter for expert dentist and doctor recognition. However, it is yet another reason why regular mouth checks at the dentist are essential, and are in no way replaced by self-inspection. But approached in the same manner as we approach other self-inspections, it can be a useful way of warding off – or at the least minimizing – the effects of dental and mouth diseases.

Chapter Two

The Dentist's Check-up

While every dentist will tell you that regular check-ups are a good thing, there are differences of opinion about how often these should be. Some dentists suggest every six months, others every year, and yet others suggest longer intervals. In reality it should depend on the age of the person and the state of the oral hygiene, gums and teeth.

Tooth decay is rampant in the first two decades of life, levels out for the next four decades, and can accelerate rapidly from then on. On the other hand the progression of gum disease accelerates as we get older. Obviously there are exceptions to this rule, but it suggests that check-ups will be for different reasons according to age. Equally children and people with a history of rampant decay, or bad gums, will benefit from more frequent check-ups. While it is tempting to add people with bad oral hygiene to this short list, most will end up being beyond dental redemption unless they improve.

Many dentists send out cards or letters telling their patients when the time has come for their check-up. Others book an appointment for the patient's next check-up at the time of the last routine visit. And yet others are so busy that they can do neither, and rely on the patient remembering – or perhaps self-examinations provoking an appointment. If you are not routinely informed about your next check-up, put an entry into your diary, planner or calendar as soon as you return from your last visit, to remind you to make a later appointment with your dentist. This is particularly important for children. The price of delay may be lost teeth.

Procedure

The dental check-up proceeds along methodical lines. The purpose is to determine the health of the mouth and teeth and whether either preventive or remedial work needs to be done, and if so what it is. The list below is based on a first examination at a new dentist. Many of the questions and actions may be unnecessary if you have been going to the dentist for some time, and he or she can refer to a lengthy dental and medical history. Although each dentist will have his or her pet order of doing things, and may place more emphasis on one factor than another, the general pattern of a dental examination is as follows:

- The dentist will need to know your name, address, age, telephone number and possibly NHS number.
- The dentist will need to know about your general health. This includes pregnancy, diabetes, heart trouble, blood pressure problems, infectious hepatitis, rheumatic fever, drug addiction, HIV status, allergies, and medication (including homeopathic or herbal) being taken or just finished. It is important that you answer completely and truthfully. Various precautions may need to be taken.

- The dentist will want to know what, if any, dental problems have brought you to the surgery – pain, sensitivity, bleeding gums or dental accidents.
- The dentist will need to know your dental history: when you last visited the dentist; any problems, such as excessive bleeding after extractions or allergic reactions; whether you prefer local or general anaesthetics, and when you last had x-rays.
- The dentist will then examine your mouth and teeth and make a record of which teeth are present or missing, if they are filled or crowned, and if there is bridge work and/or dentures. This is called *'charting'*. This is the record that the police use when they identify mutilated or decomposed bodies by their teeth.
- The dentist will use a focused light source, a mirror and a small, pointed instrument with a right-angled head (a *probe*). This will be used to check for damage to the outside of the tooth that is not immediately visible to the naked eye (roughening or softening of the outer layer of enamel), and whether there are any small ledges or gaps between existing dental work (fillings, crowns and inlays) and the teeth.
- Each time decay is found it is entered on the dentists 'chart', indicating the appropriate parts of the tooth, by the dental nurse. The dentist's instruction to the nurse may sound like gobbledegook. In fact it is very logical. With a full quota of thirty-two adult teeth, the mouth can be divided into four quarters. In each quarter, each tooth is given a number from 1 to 8, starting in the middle and working to the back. So you can have an 'upper right 3' or a 'lower left 6', etc. (see Figure 2). And each of the five surfaces of the tooth has a name. We shall cover these, their

abbreviations, and the various types of holes and fillings in Chapters 13 and 15.

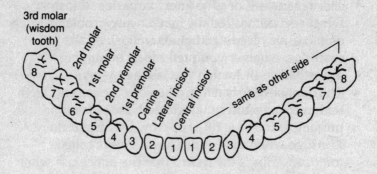

Figure 2 Names and numbers of permanent teeth

- If a dentist suspects that a tooth has died, he or she will test it by seeing whether you can feel sensation, generally by applying a very cold substance (*ethyl chloride*) or a very mild electric pulse to the tooth. If you can feel this the tooth is still alive; if not it is dead.
- The dentist will then chart any loose teeth, and measure spaces between the teeth and gums using a blunt-ended, calibrated probe. The deeper the instrument goes the worse is the gum disease and bone loss. This is called '*pocketing*'. The dentist will also check for gum bleeding. This will also be charted.
- The dentist will check for calculus deposits, the presence of plaque, and the general state of mouth and tooth hygiene, and make a survey of the general health of the gums and linings of the mouth (*mucosa*).

The dentist will also look for abscesses, small openings from chronic abscesses (*sinuses*) and ulcers.

- The dentist will examine the mouth, tongue and cheeks for signs of abnormal lumps or bumps.
- Dentures will be checked for fit, wear, cracks or damage, and bones and gums (*ridges*) for any suspicious sores, patches, ulcers or bumps.
- The dentist will spend time talking to young children, putting them at their ease, before checking their teeth, especially the permanent teeth if they are present.
- The dentist will note delayed eruption of either milk or second teeth, as well as the alignment of the jaws, crooked teeth or other factors that might need orthodontic treatment at a later date.
- At a first visit the dentist may well take x-rays. This will be for two reasons. Specific x-rays of a tooth or teeth can show what is happening inside the bone at the root end (*apex*), or determine the precise extent of bone loss around a tooth. Other x-rays, called '*bite-wings*', show whether there is decay between the teeth, and how widespread is the decay inside teeth. Pan-oral x-rays may also be taken.
- The dentist can now discuss dental problems in the context of a treatment plan, taking into account your preferences and needs. The discussion will also touch on the probable number of visits, costs and the system under which treatment will be given.
- If there is time the dentist may do a minor scaling (removal of calculus).
- The dentist may also discuss oral hygiene, and give treatment for immediate relief of urgent problems.
- The dentist may decide to refer you to a specialist dentist, or perhaps a doctor if he or she feels that

there is something in your mouth that needs specialist diagnosis or skills. This will certainly be true of unusual lumps and bumps.
- If your teeth and mouth are in good health and have been well looked after, it is possible that you may hear those magic words: 'No treatment needed.'

While the dentist obviously has responsibilities to you, the patient, it should be a reciprocal arrangement. As the patient you have certain responsibilities towards the dentist. You should always try to have a clean mouth, without food debris. If possible – and we appreciate this may not always be the case – clean your teeth shortly before attending. Stale alcohol does not smell inviting. You should always answer the questions honestly, even if this may cause embarrassment. For most of the time this is for your own protection, but in some instances it is also in the dentist's and dental staff's interests.

Chapter Three

How to Find a Dentist

Finding a dentist is both easy and difficult. It is easy to find the addresses of all the dentists in your area. But it is more difficult to find one you trust, and with whom you can feel comfortable and at home, in the absence of meaningful information. In the UK this is complicated by the fact that some people may wish to have National Health Service (NHS) treatment, but their particular area may have few dentists offering a complete NHS service. We shall explain the fee and patient payment systems in Chapter 4.

Finding NHS Treatment

The first point to realize is that a dentist in general practice is entitled to refuse, and cannot be compelled, to offer treatment to any particular person, either privately or under NHS terms. The current NHS system has decreased the numbers of general dental practitioners (GDPs) willing to provide NHS treatment. Finding the names, addresses and telephone numbers of local NHS dentists is, on the face of it, as simple as calling the local Family Health Service Authority (FHSA) in England and Wales, the local Health Board in Scotland and the

Health and Social Services Board in Northern Ireland, and asking for a list of all dentists who provide some NHS treatment. Each of these bodies is in the local telephone book.

However, it is not quite that straightforward. These lists may be less than helpful. They include all dentists who have undertaken NHS work in the previous six months, but this may have been merely a single filling or examination in what is an almost totally private sector practice. It is essential, therefore, that you ask any dentist you approach whether he or she is prepared to offer treatment under the NHS system. If the answer is 'yes', you should then find out which, if any, treatments are excluded, as many dentists do not offer to undertake all treatment on an NHS basis.

Some dentists will accept your children but not you as NHS patients. If you cannot find an NHS dentist willing to take you and your family, and you all want NHS treatment, you should contact the FHSA again. Some of them employ general practice dentists directly on a salary basis to cover for such contingencies. However, many FHSAs do not.

Other places in which you can find dentists' names and addresses are public libraries (many of which carry lists) and the local trade telephone directories – generally *Yellow Pages* or *Thomson*'s. These are the best places to find out the availability of non-NHS dentists. Local and regional papers may also carry advertisements for local dental practices. Finally a walk along the local high street or town centre should reveal several dental surgery signs.

Finding a Good Dentist

Everyone wants to find a 'good' dentist. Unfortunately, what defines 'good' for one person is irrelevant to another. It is a very personal thing. But if you work on the principle that your friends and family have similar judgements to yourself in such matters, you could do worse than follow their recommendations. However, this could lead to your receiving several suggestions. As all dentists are obliged to produce a document outlining who works in the practice and the times and types of physical access, it may be worth getting hold of several. However, there are other factors that might determine your choice.

Below, we offer a list of attributes that you may wish to take into account. On the assumption that most general practice dentists are of reasonable and similar competence, and to be registered by the General Dental Council (GDC) at one time they must have displayed such competence, you may want to consider some, or all, of the following:

- A male or female dentist. If this is of concern to you, always check the availability of either in the newer, larger, group practices.
- A sympathetic person with whom you feel comfortable.
- A talkative, chatty dentist (or a taciturn one).
- A gentle dentist who works without you noticing.
- An extremely thorough, firm dentist.
- A dentist who is good with your children.
- A surgery where a dental hygienist attends.
- A dentist who charges considerable amounts of money.

- A dentist who will always work unsocial hours to accommodate your appointments.
- A dentist who is willing to make home (domiciliary) visits.
- A dentist who speaks an appropriate language.
- Very modern surgery equipment.
- A delightful waiting room with good magazines, fish, etc.
- A dental surgery with disabled or other special access.
- A group practice or a single- or double-handed practice.
- A branch of a 'company chain' practice.
- A dentist who gives the type of anaesthesia or treatment you want. This may include hypnosis or acupuncture.

Some of these must be explained. A group practice is one where there are generally several dentists, many of whom do not work full-time. It is entirely possible that you will be treated by different dentists if you arrive in an emergency. The same tends to apply to a branch of a 'company chain' practice. Many of these work from smart shop-fronted premises with information on dental matters displayed in the window. There is a tendency for dentists who work in these practices to move on more rapidly than those in smaller practices. If you are the sort of person who needs a reassuring continuity, these are perhaps not the best places for you, although the dental standards are at least as high as anywhere else.

The FHSA (and its Scottish and Northern Irish equivalents) should be able to tell you which dental practices have disabled access, although a call to the practice itself will probably get a more up-to-date answer. People who are HIV positive, have AIDS or are hepatitis-B positive sometimes find it difficult to get dentists to treat them. Hospital HIV specialist departments and FHSA care facilities generally maintain a list of dentists who are willing to see and treat these patients.

One word of caution. It may not be wise to change dentists, unless you have lost confidence in your existing one. No two dentists will agree entirely about treatment. There are cases of what technically is called 'overprescribing', in other words performing treatments – mainly fillings – that may not have been needed, but despite publicity these are rare. (Indeed, a 1995 BBC 2 television programme suggested that there is a greater accord between dentists today about what treatment is necessary than ever before.) However, if you change dentist you may be letting yourself in for more treatment than your original dentist suggested. This is because a new dentist will not know your dental history, dental decay record (especially the rate at which your teeth decay) or the history of individual teeth. So a filling that looks stained, chipped or even slightly cracked, but which has been left like this for many years by the old dentist on the grounds that it has been performing satisfactory, may look to a new dentist as though it needs replacing as a matter of urgency. This is not to say that either the old or new one was wrong. It is just that dental opinions – like legal and medical ones – are always likely to vary.

Dental Hospitals

Dental hospitals are attached to universities, and are places where dental students are trained. They provide a full range of dental services, mostly free of charge, in specialist departments. Most of the standard work is done by students, but under the close supervision of expert tutors. The pace of treatment is slower than in general practice, but the results are generally excellent. There are, however, lengthy waiting lists for routine treatments. To get treatment you have to be referred by a dental practitioner, or attend the emergency department of the dental hospital. If there is a shortage of patients in your problem area you will be referred speedily to the appropriate department(s). Some departments, such as orthodontics, take most of their referrals from general practice or community service dentists.

These departments make up a complete range of specialist services in dedicated clinics offered by such hospitals. They may be staffed by dentists who also have their own private specialist practices. In London there is also one post-graduate teaching hospital (Eastman), which provides a similar range of services, but all by referral from your own dentist. The treatments offered here tend to be more complex.

Most large general hospitals, especially in the majority of cities and towns which have no dental hospital, will have an oral surgeon, an orthodontist, and possibly a conservationist (see Chapter 10, page 91) on staff who will treat referrals from dental practices. They also provide treatment plans and advice to local general dental practitioners. There are also emergency dental facilities should you have a haemorrhage, or perhaps a child with an acute dental infection, in the middle of the night. Some smaller hospitals with emergency departments may also have emergency dental facilities.

Community Dentistry Service

The community dentistry service was created out of the old schools dental service. It is now run and funded by District Health Authorities. Although in theory it offers a full range of dental services to children attending schools, and 'special needs' patients (generally defined as pregnant women, nursing mothers and disabled and housebound people), its main focus is the children. It is a free service, although 'special needs' patients, who in other circumstances would be eligible for NHS fees, pay for denture and bridge work. In reality this will not apply to the overwhelming number of patients. At one time, 'special needs' included people who were unable to get NHS dental treatment in their area. However, the current NHS market system no longer allows the community dental service to treat people in this predicament.

Most FHSAs run clinics and surgeries that have access for disabled people, and lifts when necessary. For those who cannot even get to the surgery, the service also provides a full domiciliary service for the housebound. Some clinics provide a service to those with a phobia of dental surgeries. Community dentists also staff the school 'dental screening' system. This aims to examine each schoolchild a minimum of three times in their school career. Some community dental service patients come from these check-ups, others are referred by social workers, while others who are disabled and/or have gross decay may be referred by general practitioners.

Other Dental Service Providers

The FHSA (and the Scottish and Northern Irish equivalents) are charged with the provision of NHS dental facilities for all those who need them. This means that they have to ensure that there are specialist NHS orthodontists and general practitioners in each area. However, if there is a significant shortfall of NHS general practitioners, some FHSAs employ salaried general practitioner dentists to take up the slack. While much of the treatment is free (not dentures, crowns or bridges for those eligible to pay for them), a change in NHS regulations is likely to make charges for all treatments compulsory for those eligible to pay. University student dental departments were originally put in place to treat students, especially those living away from home. However, they now take patients from faculties as well, and, as most now have to be self-funding, some also act as general dental practices.

Dental Treatment Abroad

It is unlikely that you will need routine dental treatment on a trip abroad, unless you are away for a very considerable period. The need for emergency treatment is, however, by no means unknown, and finding a dentist can prove to be a nightmare of Elm Street proportions. Package tour couriers can generally point you towards a dentist who speaks some English, and hotel desks can also point you in the right direction, although this service may vary. Whether you have broken a tooth, crown or bridge, lost a denture or just have a toothache, you should look for short-term emergency treatment and have it completed by your own dentist on return.

We shall cover the costs for treatment abroad in Chapter 4, but the rule of thumb is that you should be prepared to pay for treatment on the spot, even if some fees may be reimbursed later. To get reimbursed, however, you should be as prepared as a scout and as tenacious as a bulldog when it comes to hunting and filling in forms.

Chapter Four

Paying for the Treatment

Dental treatment can be free and it can be extremely
expensive. One hospital consultant was shown a £58,000
estimate submitted to a patient for what is known as
a 'full mouth rehabilitation'. Put in a proper context
this price would be far less than this particular patient
would normally pay for a new car. And in the greater
scheme of things your mouth is far more valuable, and
considerably less replaceable, than any car.

However, given prices at that level, it is a relief to
report that the majority of UK dental treatment is still
under NHS auspices. But the current method of providing these dental services is not only relatively new,
it is also under intermittent threat of change, and social
security and health service systems are probably at even
greater risk of radical change. So everything in this
chapter must be qualified by 'at the time of writing'.
And at this time only 50 per cent of all dentists offer a
complete NHS service, and – as most of you who live
there know without us telling you – this falls dramatically to around 30 per cent in parts of southern England.
This is because, while NHS fees are the same all over
the country, nearly every single practice overhead costs
more in the south.

The health care offered under the NHS general dental
practice service falls into three categories. In each of

these, there will be a written agreement between the patient and the dentist.

1. Continuing care for under 18-year-olds (under 19-year-olds in full-time education). This is free for the patient. Dentists get a flat capitation fee per patient and an annual continuing care fee. For these fees, dentists are expected to make the youngsters dentally fit, and then keep them dentally fit. Clearly young people with poor oral hygiene (and probably rampant decay and bad gums) are not a good commercial prospect for the dentist, and could be at some risk of not having the agreement renewed at its annual review.

2. Continuing care for adults. This agreement is based on a two-year arrangement. The patient pays 80 per cent of the NHS scale of fees up to a maximum of £300 per course of treatment. (If the total cost of treatment is higher than £200 the dentist will need approval of the FHSA, and treatment will be delayed.) The NHS scale of fees is based on the piecework concept (except for the under 18-year-olds where the dentist is not paid a fee for any work at all). Some people are exempt from any charges. These are:

    a. pregnant women and nursing mothers (women who have had a baby in the preceding twelve months);

    b. people receiving income support, family credit and disability working allowance. The dentist gets an extremely modest cash sum to keep an adult registered as a patient for the two-year period. Short of a cataclysmic destruction of the patient–dentist relationship

– or more probably the dentist deciding to stop NHS treatments altogether – there is no reason why the registration should not be maintained. However, patients may change their dentist as and when they please.

3. The third category is 'occasional treatment'. Occasional treatment is the UK equivalent of looking for a foreign dentist. People having this sort of treatment may be working away from home, or on a UK holiday. However, dentists are not allowed to offer a full range of NHS treatment under this system, where again the patient pays 80 per cent of the NHS fee scale.

Every new person who signs an agreement for continuing care is entitled to a treatment plan from the dentist explaining what treatment is needed and what it will cost, unless only minimal treatment is needed. At the time of writing, a person whose treatment is under NHS auspices will pay £4 for a check-up, just over £4 for a small filling, almost £6.50 for a simple scale and polish and instructions in oral hygiene and only just over £17 for a single-canal root-filling on an incisor. Compared with the estimate at the start of this chapter these are unmistakable bargains. And it is worth keeping in mind that the more regularly you pay the £4 for the check-up, the less likely it is that you will have to spend considerable amounts of money on the more expensive treatments at a later date. You should always pay the dentist. Although it generally takes three months' notice for a dentist to terminate a continuing care agreement, this can be done immediately if the fees are not paid. Indeed, a dentist is entitled to ask for the entire cost of treatment at the first visit. Dentists should also arrange for out-of-hours emergency treatment for their patients on the NHS continuing care list. Some operate a cooperative rota; others have come to an arrangement with the local general hospital to provide this service.

We have already mentioned the four free treatment centres: dental teaching hospitals, general hospitals, salaried general dental practitioners and the community dental service. (The latter two generally only treat patients who would be exempt from NHS payments anyway.) In marked contrast to these is the private dental sector. Most general practice dentists will do some private work if they are asked to do so. Some, however, will do only private work, and most dentists specializing in a specific field will only work privately.

It is possible to mix NHS and private treatment in a single course of treatment. For example, a dentist may offer extractions and fillings on an NHS basis, but make the subsequent partial dentures on a private basis. However, the dentist must not only make such a proposal clear at the initial stages in the treatment plan, but also not intimate that certain treatments are unavailable on NHS terms, unless of course they genuinely are not available.

All private sector dentistry is based on either piecework or the time taken to perform the treatment. The longer and more complicated the treatment the higher the cost. Some fees explicitly pay both the dentist and the technician who makes the denture, crown or bridge work. The level of fees depends on which part of the country the dentist is in. Giving a comparative example with the NHS, an incisor root filling will cost between £55 and £180, and a small filling between £18 and £60.

As with medicine and surgery, where fees are so high that they are well beyond the pockets of many people, insurance schemes have entered the market to ease the burden. However, they differ from the standard medical insurance where the consumer chooses from a list of hospitals, pays the bills and is reimbursed. Denplan, one of the older dental insurance schemes, signs up the dentists, not the patients. People opt for the scheme at their dentist, but pay their monthly premiums to Denplan, which then reimburses the dentist for work done according to which scale of fees they are on. The scale is based on the patient's original dental condition – the worse it is the higher the monthly payment. Patients also pay any laboratory fees incurred. In effect, Denplan is less an insurance scheme than a prepayment budget scheme for continuing dental treatment (or health) where a small part of the monthly payment also buys insurance for emergency and accident cover. Other dental 'insurance' schemes, such as BUPA, work in the same general way. There are generally exclusions, such as prolonged orthodontic treatment for children, or implant work. Some ordinary medical insurance policies will pay for some dental work, notably the surgical extraction of wisdom teeth.

Payment for dental treatment abroad falls into two categories. European Union (EU) countries work with EU form E111 to offer free (not at time of use) or reduced cost emergency treatment. Most other countries do not. Form E111 can be obtained, along with an explanatory leaflet T5 'Health Advice for Travellers', from post offices. This leaflet explains, in some detail, which offices to go to in each of the EU countries to collect the appropriate forms to make a claim for the reimbursement of dental emergency fees. It also explains what you need to take with you. Generally this will be a passport, your NHS card and the E111 form. To be frank it does not sound easy, unless you are an expert form-filler, and it has to be wondered how many people actually travel with the latter two items about their person.

The leaflet also supplies details of countries outside the EU with reciprocal health care agreements with the UK. Few of these offer dental services. The leaflet is worth keeping, however, for its wider medical care information. Most countries with some form of socialized medicine run their basic dental services on a rebate system. You pay the dentist and then receive a percentage rebate at a later date. This is a form of state insurance scheme. Private insurance schemes are also common in the EU. In the United States a novel scheme that puts the emphasis on prevention is run by a handful of US companies for employees and ex-employees. They pay a minimum sum every six months to have a full check-up. Providing they continue to do this, all subsequent treatment is free. This is a proper preventive medical service, with a market incentive to take part.

Chapter Five

Prevention –
Always Better than Cure

Recent research from Sweden suggests very strongly that our dental health is literally in our own hands. Diseases of teeth and gums could be a thing of the past if we cleaned our teeth better and more frequently. However, the routine needed for perfection is beyond the discipline, let alone the patience, of most people. In the real world other factors such as a job, family and socializing will always reduce the time available to reach dental nirvana. However, this does not mean that we cannot improve both our mouth hygiene and our diet so that we minimize, if not banish, tooth decay and gum disease.

Most people want their teeth to look good, so they clean them. They also use mouthwashes to sweeten the breath. It is a huge commercial market. In recent years traditional toothpastes have been replaced by new flavours and products aimed at different sections of the teeth-cleaning public. People with sensitive teeth, people bothered by plaque or gum trouble, people who want whiter teeth and troubled smokers are all catered for. We spend a lot of money on these products, yet the general standard of teeth cleaning leaves a lot to be desired. It tends to be superficial. It needs to be thorough.

We came across plaque at the beginning of the book. In mouth terms it is an assassin first class – the 'Jackal' of the dentition. But it is aided and abetted in its work of destruction by foodstuffs and drinks that are converted into acids in plaque. So the prevention of tooth decay and gum disease depends on a double-pronged defence. The first prong is to remove plaque before it has a chance to do any damage, and the second is to cut down on acid-generating food and drinks.

Plaque is removed by the proper cleaning of teeth. Indeed, the major purpose of teeth cleaning is to get rid of plaque, not to remove bits of food, or even to have a sparkling smile, although this may be a delightful by-product of good cleaning. It is worth repeating that the main thing to remember about cleaning teeth is that every tooth has five surfaces, and each surface should be cleaned. Just using a toothbrush, be it ordinary or electric, can only clean the front, the back and the tips and tops. It cannot clean between the teeth. And this is where so much dental trouble starts, and finishes.

Not only are there increasing numbers of toothpastes and mouthwashes on the market, there are also various implements with which you can clean your teeth. Before moving on to actual tooth and mouth cleaning, we outline the more common available implements:

- toothbrushes with heads of various sizes and angles
- electric toothbrushes
- interdental (bottle) brushes
- medicated gum massage sticks
- dental floss
- water picks
- mouthwashes

Toothbrushes

The key thing about choosing a toothbrush is that it should be capable of cleaning all the reachable tooth surfaces in your mouth. This argues for a smaller, rather than larger brush-head. Straight-handled toothbrushes suit some people; kinkily-handled ones suit others. Which you prefer depends partly on the shape of your mouth and partly on the ability of your hands and wrists to manipulate the head of the brush to the remoter back corners of your mouth. The important thing is that it must do the work for you.

Soft-bristle brushes are not really capable of removing plaque; they merely smear it over the surface of the teeth. On the other hand, very hard bristles can act like wire-wool on the gums, or indeed the teeth. A medium-hard, firm-bristled toothbrush is the best for both teeth and gums. Organic bristles, as opposed to nylon or other synthetic material, tend to become too soft, and wear out very quickly. As they also take a long time to dry out they also have a tendency to harbour bacteria. This is one of those occasions when 'artificial' appears to be preferable to 'natural'. It is also important to change your toothbrush regularly, as floppy, straggly bristles are just not up to plaque removal.

Electric toothbrushes

Modern electric toothbrushes have a rechargeable electric motor driving a standard or rotary head. Compared with an ordinary toothbrush they are very expensive; indeed an under-used argument for buying an electric toothbrush is that it costs so much that you feel you have to use it properly to justify the investment. And used properly it is very efficient.

Interdental brushes

Also called 'bottle' brushes. They have a small, single-spiral, tapered brush-head built around a wire core, which is at a right-angle to the handle. Some have a head at either end of the handle, and many brushes have detachable heads to cut the cost of replacement, which has to be frequent. There are also single tufted interspace brushes. Both are designed to clean between the teeth (the interdental areas). In other words they clean the fourth and fifth surfaces of the teeth, as do the following two products.

Medicated gum massage sticks

These are small pieces of wood, triangular in cross-section, one or both ends of which have been tapered along one surface to make a sharpish wedge. They may be medicated and are intended to clean away the plaque from the gums and between the teeth. They are often sold under proprietary labels in packet form, like books of matches. They can also have fluoride additives.

Dental floss and tape

Floss is a thin twine-like cord that is manipulated between the teeth. Again it is designed to clean away the plaque from the gums and between the teeth. It comes in reels or boxes and can be waxed or unwaxed. Dental tape, which is becoming more popular, is flatter and wider and has similar uses. Furryfloss (also known as superfloss) may also be used, especially to clean under sections of bridge work. Both floss and tape can be bought with added fluoride.

Water picks
These are electrically driven appliances that direct a variable strength jet of water. There are various size nozzles for access to between the teeth, and mouthwash can be added to the water if required.

Mouthwashes
Most mouthwashes promise to give sweet breath. While many have disappointing dental results – not to mention downright counterproductive high acidity, which could actually lead to increased tooth decay – those containing *chlorhexidine* help to control gum disease and control inflammation under dentures. As they have a demonstrable anti-plaque effect they are also of use for the young, the elderly and anyone else who is caries prone. They may also be bought in spray form, and in both forms aid the healing of mouth ulcers. Many mouthwashes contain added fluoride.

Teeth Cleaning

If only cleaning your teeth was a more exciting way to spend time we would not have to write this section. It is, however, one of those activities that we have to do, rather than like to do (similar to filling a car with petrol), and where time also plays funny tricks on us. Every twenty seconds spent cleaning your teeth feels like at least one minute. And you need to spend a good three minutes cleaning them once, but preferably twice, every day.

Most of us clean our teeth before or just after

breakfast and/or just before bedtime. And most of us are not at our brightest at either of these times. So it is all too easy to start cleaning your teeth, then letting the mind wander over your plans for the day, or perhaps mulling over what actually happened. Unfortunately, at the end of scrubbing away for about a minute, you haven't a clue whether you have cleaned your entire mouth or just a few teeth. It may sound pretentious, but teeth cleaning requires some concentration. We need a mechanism that allows us to clean our teeth properly and purposefully each time.

The trick of good teeth cleaning is to adopt a routine that covers every surface of every single tooth. Both parts of this are important – the conscious cleaning of each surface of each tooth and the routine that enables you to do this on some form of autopilot. Stick to a settled route around the mouth. If you are right-handed you may want to start on the back molar on the upper left side. First brush the surface next to the cheek, then the biting surface and then the surface on the inside. Working towards the centre, repeat this with each tooth until you reach the middle. Then go through the same routine with the bottom left teeth. Repeat these actions for the teeth on the right-hand side.

The actual route is up to you. You may prefer to clean all the top teeth first, then the bottom ones, or the inside of all the top teeth and then their outside surfaces. It does not matter providing the routine enables you to clean all the teeth, on all the reachable surfaces, all the time, every time.

The intention is to remove all the plaque. Plaque is a complex mixture. It is formed by a species of bacterium, the streptococcus. In other circumstances this can give us the classic sore throat. Here it sticks to the outer surfaces of teeth and forms a slightly sticky web that attracts other substances, salivary proteins and other bacteria. Sadly for us this process does not take long. About 6 hours after cleaning your teeth, they will be covered with plaque again, even if you have not eaten.

The actual process of cleaning doesn't need a great deal of toothpaste, certainly not as much as the toothpaste advertisements would have you believe. The classic description is 'pea-sized', which is the maximum of fluoride toothpaste to be used by a child under the age of 7. (N.B. Only use children's toothpaste for children under 7 years of age, because it contains only half the optimum level of fluoride additive.) While on this topic it is worth repeating that the widespread use of toothpastes with added fluoride appear to have reduced tooth decay very substantially. They have done this by strengthening the enamel layer of the tooth, rather like adding super-toughened Chobham armour to a battle-tank. There are also toothpastes that promise to act against plaque and calculus deposits, but with less proven effects. However, a new breed of toothpastes with more claims to being effective are now being developed (see Chapter 14).

When cleaning teeth, the toothbrush should be used so that its head is held at a 45 degree angle to the tooth, not the full face of the bristles. This is especially important when cleaning at the junction of the tooth and gum, and where the tooth meets the one next to it, because it allows the brush to reach the plaque deposits that occur there (see Figure 3 below).

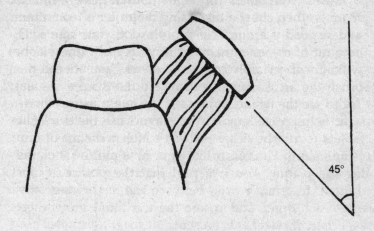

Figure 3 Correct brushing angle for reaching plaque deposits

You should brush in small circular scrubbing move-ments. Take care not to damage your gums or the teeth next to the gums by excessively strenuous brushing. Electric toothbrushes are just held against the tooth surfaces, and moved slowly along. Done properly you should brush away all the plaque.

But how do you know if you have removed the plaque totally? After all, it is not highly visible, unless it has been allowed to collect for a few days. The answer lies in tablets called 'disclosing tablets' that you buy from the chemist. (As these are only vegetable dyes, it might be cheaper to make your own 'disclosing solution' from a generic vegetable dye.) They are either a vivid 'raspberry lolly' red or a violent blue. The dye sticks to plaque, but not to a clean tooth. You avoid staining your lips by smearing them with Vaseline before using the tablets; in any event the stain wears off quickly.

Clean your teeth in your normal absent-minded manner, then chew a disclosing tablet for a full minute, and swoosh it around the mouth with your saliva. The amount of colour remaining on your teeth (the plaque) will almost certainly come as a shock. You should then brush the areas of the teeth where the plaque remains. Try to see the inside surfaces of the teeth: using a bright light helps considerably. You should use the disclosing tablets regularly, either before or after the start of your cleaning, until it is clear that your new routine is removing the plaque. You will find that the plaque is most difficult to remove from between the teeth where they meet each other, and where the teeth and gums meet, especially if calculus is present.

Let us suppose that you have all thirty-two teeth. With three sides to clean on each tooth this means that even if you spend as little as 1 second per side it would take you 1½ minutes to clean them all. But proper removal of plaque will take longer than this, so even when practice has made perfect you are probably looking at a minimum of 3 minutes basic cleaning time.

Cleaning the Fourth and Fifth Surfaces

But this is far from the entire story. You still have to clean those fourth and fifth surfaces between the teeth. This is where you have a choice. You can either use dental floss, the interdental brush, or perhaps the medicated gum massage sticks.

Flossing

Trying to learn how to floss by reading a book is as un-rewarding to the reader as listening to a juggler on the radio. There is something missing. In reality a video, or a personal demonstration, is needed. The simple way of flossing is to hold the floss between two fingers (or wind it around them), hold it taught and then push it (up or down) between two teeth and into the space between the gum and tooth (if it exists). It is then pulled backwards and forwards, up and down along the side of the adjacent teeth. This dislodges food debris and removes plaque. With practice, floss can be inserted between almost all teeth, despite the initial feeling that some teeth are too close together. As with ordinary cleaning a routine needs to be established so as not to miss the spaces between some teeth.

Unfortunately, as dental floss is not easy to use, many people become discouraged by their failure. However, there are products on the market intended to help. They look like miniature catapults with the floss stretched across the two prongs of the Y acting as the fingers, but you only have to hold one stem. Even so, expert instruction will be needed to get the angles required for optimal cleaning between the back teeth. If you are keen to try the procedure we suggest you ask your dentist to arrange a demonstration for you. Expert flossing will always keep those fourth and fifth surfaces free from plaque.

Medicated Gum-Massage Sticks

Medicated gum-massage sticks are inserted horizontally between the teeth from the outer surface and moved backwards and forwards between the teeth. They both massage the gum where two teeth touch each other and clean plaque away from the inside (fourth and fifth) surfaces of the teeth and the gums. They need to be used with determination, although this may be at the cost of many broken sticks.

Bottle Brushes

Many people find bottle brushes the easiest to use of all the fourth and fifth surface cleaners. The tiny white Christmas-tree-shaped head is pushed horizontally between the teeth. The bristles should be touching the teeth either side (and resting on the gum between the teeth). It is pushed to-and-fro with some vigour. If there is a large gap between the teeth, one side should be cleaned, then the brush moved to the other side. You should try to insert the brush from the inner surface of the tooth, as well as from the outer surface, so removing all the plaque. The same procedure applies to single-tufted interspace brushes.

If you want healthy teeth and gums, cleaning between the teeth should be part of your daily routine. Plaque creates the gum troubles that lead to loose teeth, and you must clear it away. You may get bleeding and a nasty smell from this form of cleaning. The more inflamed (and unhealthier) the gum the more easily it bleeds. The smell comes from either plaque, decomposing food, infection, or some combination of them. Regular use of floss, sticks or bottle brushes should lessen both the bleeding and smell over time. However, if your gums bleed or you have a continual bad taste in your mouth, you should consult your dentist.

Other Products

Water-picks

Water-picks use a jet of high-pressure water directed at the teeth and gums. The force is insufficient to dislodge much, if any, plaque. However, they are good at clearing food debris and making the mouth feel fresh.

Mouthwashes

Although many mouthwashes are advertised as plaque-removing or neutralizing most are not in contact with the teeth for long enough to have a great effect. Unfortunately, a mouth that feels clean is not necessarily one that *is* clean. Chlorhexidine mouthwash (or gel) does have some effect in 'dissolving' plaque. However, it has the disadvantage of staining plaque a brownish colour, making it appear that the teeth are dirty. However, new mouthwashes and a chlorhexidine-based toothpaste are more dilute, and less staining. Proper cleaning, however, is still the key. Ultimately, you will know that you are cleaning properly when your gums don't bleed and you have clear dental check-ups.

Cleaning Crowns, Bridges and Dentures

We shall deal with cleaning children's teeth in Chapter 6, so we are left with cleaning around crowns, bridges and dentures. It is important to clean very thoroughly around teeth that have been crowned or where bridge work is in place. This is because, with the best will in the world, the seal between the stump of the tooth and the crown cannot be perfect, and you really want to avoid any decay starting. Decay under a crown can be painful, inconvenient and ultimately expensive. You also want to avoid food getting trapped, or plaque building up, between bridges and the gums and adjacent teeth, as this can lead to gum trouble as well as decay. This cleaning is done in the same way as described above, but perhaps with more use of floss and the bottle brush.

Dentures should also be cleaned to rid them of plaque and especially calculus. You should give all dentures a good scrub with a stiff brush at least once a day. This is a necessary addition to the rinse and soak you give them in a proprietary denture-cleansing solution.

Diet

As we have already suggested, keeping plaque at bay is only half the solution. Minimizing your intake of food and drink that can break down to form acids in the mouth is the other. In very simplified terms this is because these foods and plaque combine to form acids in contact with the surface of the teeth. These are strong enough to 'eat' through the hard, outer enamel layer of the tooth. Once this has been accomplished, the bacteria in the plaque enter the softer parts of the tooth (the dentine) and decay begins in earnest (see Figure 4)

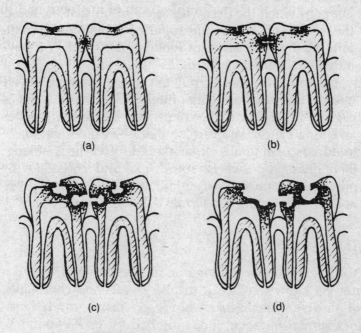

(a) (b)

(c) (d)

Figure 4 Progression of decay: (a) acids attacking outer enamel;
(b) bacteria starting to destroy the underlying dentine; (c) decay spreading
inside tooth; (d) unsupported area of tooth broken off

Figure 4a shows two back teeth where acids are attacking the outer enamel and eating it away, both on the biting surfaces and between the teeth. By the time we reach Figure 4b the acids have made holes in the enamel and bacteria have moved inside the tooth and are starting to destroy the underlying dentine. This is decay (dental caries). In Figure 4c the decay has spread inside the tooth, even though the holes on the biting surfaces may look small. What is worse is that the holes between the teeth will still be out of view. Figure 4d shows what happens when the decay has gone so far that the top of the tooth is effectively unsupported (even though to the untrained eye it may not look terrible) and you have bitten into something hard.

Basically, and not to put too fine a point on it, we need to minimize our sugar intake. Clearly this is not as easy as it sounds. If the connection between cigarettes and lung cancer and cardiac diseases cannot persuade hundreds of millions of smokers to give up smoking, then giving up sweets, soft-drinks and chocolates to protect teeth must be an uphill struggle. After all, it is not such a dramatically terminal disincentive.

The Sweet Tooth

You must have been living on another planet if you do not yet know that sweet drinks, sweets and chocolates of all descriptions, cakes, buns, ice-creams, candy-floss and similar fattening foods are bad for both children's teeth and your own. So it is probably not worth a lot of time and trouble trying to persuade you that stopping or rationing these to children is a good thing. You all know this already. But doing something about it in the face of children's stratagems is quite another matter. You cannot isolate children entirely. What with sweets at supermarket check-outs, television sweet advertising, doting grandparents, and friends apparently getting unlimited quantities of them, the substitution of carrots for Smarties is likely to be as welcome as extra homework. However, sugar-free chewing gum, such as Orbit and Endekay, can be used as substitutes for sugar-rich sweets. With care, sweet rationing is possible. How you do this is a matter for you and your children – you know their strengths and weaknesses, but incentives often seem better than penalties.

This is not only a matter that concerns children, however. There is also your own intake of sweets to worry about. Self-discipline is the key. It may help you to concentrate on the slimming potential of giving up sugary foods and drinks, from a health and an attractiveness point of view. However, there are less obvious (and less well-known) foods and drinks that also have bad tooth-decay effects.

Most sugars break down with plaque to form acids in the mouth. This means any food or drink with sugar in it. If you read the labelling on many tinned or other packaged products, you may be surprised at the large numbers that contain one sugar or another. This is the first important point. There are many forms of sugar, and the labels often use their technical names. So if you did not know that fructose was a sugar, you might have thought that the fizzy drink you were drinking was sugar-free. If you are a determined content label reader you should be looking for 'glucose', 'sucrose', 'lactose', 'fructose', and any longer word that has one of these four in it, such as 'iso-sucrose'.

Fruit is good for you, and not long ago it was thought that apples were also good for the teeth. Indeed, there was a time when dentists had pictures of apples in their surgeries, with a caption urging children to eat them. Now it is recognized that they too contain tooth-harmful sugars, as do most other fruits. However, they are not as harmful as the mainstream glucose and sucrose, and most certainly not harmful enough to stop eating fruit.

While you would probably expect tinned peaches in syrup to be high in sugars, it may surprise you to know that most tinned soups, baked beans, spaghetti, ravioli, meat and vegetarian stews and many tinned vegetables also contain added sugar, as do nearly all the proprietary pickles, ketchups and sauces on the supermarket shelves. Indeed, in the tinned and bottled area it is difficult to avoid sugars altogether.

Although milk has a high calcium and Vitamin D content, and therefore is good for teeth and bones, it too has a high sugar content. Colas, juices and other soft drinks also contain sugars, even when they claim to have no added sugar. And fizzy drinks, because they contain acids, are worse for the teeth than still drinks. It would also appear that vegetarian foodstuffs are often worse for the teeth than other foods because they tend to be accompanied by a higher than average amount of sugars and pickles to lend more taste.

Comforters should not be dipped in milk or sweet syrupy substances such as rose-hip syrup or honey, and babies' bottles should have water rather than juices in them as often as possible. Try not to keep a stock of sugary food and drink in the home, and if possible do not take the children with you to supermarkets or food shops. Sugars are not the only substances that break down to form acids in the plaque. Some other refined carbohydrates are very bad for the teeth. Indeed, some maize products used to make munchy snacks are as *cariogenic* (causing decay) as any sweet. While other foods can break down to create acids – bread, for example – the amounts needed to be eaten are so large for tooth damage to occur as to not constitute a real dental danger. And while citrus fruits, pickles and acids such as vinegar can erode teeth, for most people they make an existing problem worse, rather than create the problem in the first instance. For nearly all dental and medical researchers, sugars are the major suspect in tooth decay.

Timing

It is not only unhealthy to avoid all sugars, it is well nigh impossible (diabetics have this problem). So what can we do about tooth decay? The first thing is that we need some rules to try to minimize sugar damage, especially in young children. It can be done. The first thing to remember is that it is not only what you eat but when you eat it. So the first point is the timing of sugar intake. The acid level of plaque rises to a peak in 20 minutes, and takes a full 30 minutes to return to normal. If you keep snacking between meals there is a constantly high acid level, and constantly high rate of tooth destruction. But, for example, if a cola is drunk with a meal, or a jam sandwich with the rest of tea, there is only one danger period of up to 50 minutes for all the food and drink. So always try to eat sweets or other sugary foods or drinks at normal meal times.

We should try to be sensible about eating and drinking. It is more than useful that healthy eating, in terms of avoiding obesity and heart problems, corresponds precisely with dentally healthy eating. Basically this means a balanced diet. Many dentists recommend eating savoury rather than sweet snacks (especially for children), and some crunchy foods such as celery and carrots, which may have a marginal cleaning effect. Overall, however, it is a matter of avoiding or minimizing your intake of the tooth- and gum-damaging foods and drinks, rather than seeking out dentally beneficial foods.

We can also try to clear food from the mouth immediately after eating or drinking, to avoid acid production in the plaque, but this is often impracticable, especially in the workplace. You can, however, chew sugar-free gum after a meal. This stimulates the production of saliva. Saliva is alkaline and helps neutralize the acids on the teeth.

If you look after your teeth properly there is no reason why you should not keep them all of your life. Clean plaque away as often and thoroughly as possible and you will have healthy teeth and gums, whatever you eat.

Part Two

Facts about the Mouth

Chapter Six

Babies and Young Children (up to 7 Years)

Teething

A baby's milk teeth are starting to form in the embryo after about six weeks. Some second teeth also start to form before birth. By the time a baby is born the crowns of all of its milk teeth are starting to harden *(calcify)*. They are, however, except in extremely rare cases, safely locked away in the bone beneath the gums – safely, because breast-feeding a baby with teeth could prove to be a painful process.

Babies have twenty milk teeth (see Figure 5). To distinguish them from adult teeth, which are numbered, dentists label them 'a', 'b', 'c', 'd' and 'e' for each quarter of the mouth, with 'a' starting in the middle and moving to the back for the 'e'.

It is not surprising that babies get irritable when teething. It must be a painful business. After all, the teeth have to break through the gum, which gets swollen and tender. There is considerable dribbling, hand biting, and much bad temper. As a result, parents also tend to get irritable. But it is worth noting that teething does not cause prolonged vomiting or high temperatures, convulsions or other severe medical

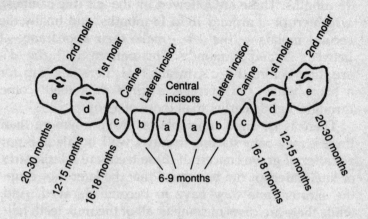

Figure 5 Names, letters and eruption dates of milk teeth

conditions. Should these occur, consult your doctor.

Proprietary teething gels are available from chemists, but none has the soothing power of the Victorian powders, which, believe it or not, contained morphine. Apart from keeping the baby clean and comfortable with the soothing gels and Calpol, and providing a teething ring, there is little that can be done. The only consolation is that it does not last long, and that the worst problems are the earliest ones, when the baby cannot talk or move around to take its mind of its predicament.

The first teeth start to poke through at between 6 and 9 months (see Figure 5 above). They start with the 'a's and then the 'b's – these are called the *incisors*. The lower teeth almost always emerge first. There is then a relatively long wait before the next milk teeth – the 'd's (the first molars) – come through at between 12 months and 15 months. These are followed by the 'c's (the canines), which erupt at around 16 to 18 months, and finally the second molars – the 'e's – make their appearance at between 20 and 30 months. This pattern, with the 'd's erupting before the 'c's, means that there is a gap for a short while. On average, a girl's milk teeth come through slightly earlier than those of a boy.

There is no rigid timetable or order, anymore than there is for a baby starting to crawl, walk or talk. It is not a matter of grave concern if these teeth are a little early or late. Indeed it can be argued that the later they erupt the shorter time they have to become decayed. And while there are cases of some or all of the milk teeth failing to appear, these are few and far between. But should this seem to be happening a dentist should be consulted to find out whether there are any milk teeth at all inside the jaw-bones, and what the status of the adult teeth in the jaws may be.

Milk Teeth

While a mother's healthy, balanced, calcium-rich diet will help the proper formation of the baby's teeth and bones, problems with the appearance or structure of milk teeth are more to do with inherited factors and, very occasionally, an illness of the mother or infant. There is a rare condition where the enamel (and sometimes dentine) of both the milk and permanent teeth does not form properly. The teeth can be very unsightly with random patches of white enamel on yellowish dentine. Some diseases, such as neonatal jaundice or porphyria, can cause discoloration, as can the heavy use of the antibiotic tetracycline, but these are becoming rarer with medical advances. People living in high fluoride areas may also get mottled teeth, a condition called *'fluorosis'*.

Milk teeth are not only necessary for eating, they also act as a guide for the position of the second teeth, as well as helping in the formation and alignment of the bones of the jaws. If this is not incentive enough for keeping them, then the thorough teasing children dish out to others who have perceptible differences – and gaps where the teeth should be is a very perceptible difference – should clinch the argument. This means that it is important to keep milk teeth healthy to avoid extractions.

Many children suck their thumb or fingers at a young age, although, as we shall see in Chapter 7, this habit can last somewhat longer. Although the sucking pressure can 'pull' the front teeth forward slightly, this is of little consequence for the milk teeth, which are shed. Using pacifiers or dummies does not seem to have quite the same level of 'pull'. Although the malpositioning of milk teeth is not generally serious and should not require treatment, it may be that the upper and lower jaws are not developing equally. If this is so, consult your dentist.

Diet

Parents have a crucial role. As we have already suggested, comforters and bottles should be totally free of milky, syrupy or sweet substances as these 'dissolve' the front milk teeth at an incredible speed, leaving behind little more than blackened stumps. Indeed, try to wean babies off bottles at an early age. An empty comforter causes no problems, and still offers a great deal of comfort. Sugars should be kept out of the diet as much as possible, as the taste for sweet things is acquired early in life rather than inborn. This will help avoid a 'sugar dependency' in later life. It is also well worth checking the contents of baby foods to avoid those with sugars, and checking medicines, especially cough syrups, for sugar content with the doctor. We must repeat, however, that with sugars the problem is not so much the quantity but *when* you have them. **Meal times only** should be the rule.

Teeth Cleaning

The other element of tooth protection, plaque removal, should start as early as possible. Initially clean around the incisor teeth with a cotton wool bud or a small baby's toothbrush, with only a tiny smidgen of toothpaste. But as the baby develops hand-to-eye coordination it is a good idea to give it a small toothbrush to play with at bath time, providing always that you also clean the teeth properly. Do remember to clean both the inside and outside of the teeth. An adult cleaning a child's teeth at night is not an optional task. Like cleaning the face it *has* to be done, and is best accomplished by standing behind the small child, in the way that the dentist works from behind you in the surgery.

Using a fluoride toothpaste is always a good idea, providing it is only a smear until the child is capable of spitting it out rather than swallowing it. There have been cases of small children swallowing too much, and getting fluoridized mottled teeth. Always keep toothpaste out of the reach of children, as they have a habit of eating it given half a chance. By the age of 6 or 7 most children should be able to clean their teeth adequately, even if the results still have to be checked by adults.

Fluoride can enter the tooth in two other ways. It occurs naturally in the water in some places in the UK, where it has been known to create the mottled teeth referred to above. It can also be added to the public water supply, as it has been in the West Midlands. Fluoride can also be administered personally in the form of tablets or drops. The tablets, which have pleasant flavours, are either crunched or allowed to dissolve, the drops are added to water. Children should *not* use either of these if they are also using fluoride toothpaste – it must be one or the other.

Although these fluoride additives not only protect teeth against decay but also repair very slightly decayed areas of tooth, they should only be used after consultation with your dentist or doctor. And you must always check on the local water supply to find the level of fluoride before embarking on a personal dosage course. You should not use them if the water contains more than 5 parts fluoride per million. And, if the family drinks a considerable amount of bottled water, the contents ought to be scrutinized for fluoride levels as well. In any event the drops should not be used until the baby is over 6 months old, and the tablets delayed until the child is over 2 years old, and again neither of them should be used if the child is already using fluoride toothpaste.

Permanent Teeth

The first permanent tooth to come through is most often at the back, behind the last milk tooth – the 'e'. This happens at 6–7 years old. The tooth is called a *molar* tooth. It is also called the '6' by the dentist. (This is not because of the age of eruption but because it is the sixth tooth from the middle towards the back of the mouth.) The milk teeth start falling out from the front incisors – 'a's then 'b's. The roots of these teeth get shorter, almost eaten away, as the permanent teeth edge down (or up) above or below them. This is why they get so loose that you can wobble them out with your fingers, and the 'tooth fairy' then takes its toll of your purse.

From time to time a milk tooth lingers on in very loose fashion, while the permanent tooth visibly lurks behind it. While this is unlikely to cause any permanent harm it can be very irritating, both to the child itself, and because of the grimaces and sounds of the tongue playing with it, to its parents. So if you, or the child, cannot loosen it sufficiently for it to shed naturally, pop along to the dentist, who will remove it.

The Dentist

It is never too early to take a child to the dentist. This may not be for treatment, or even for a proper examination. It is merely to acclimatize the child, to show that the dental surgery is not a place to fear, indeed that it can seem to be a pleasant place to visit. It is also wise to build up a friendly relationship between the dentist and the child. So try not to take the baby if you are likely to show symptoms of distress or fear, let someone who is more relaxed take the baby along.

Treatments

Although it is possible to apply fluoride (or sealants) to the surface of children's teeth, this is not done to the milk teeth. Milk teeth, however, become decayed in precisely the same way as permanent teeth. Indeed, decay often spreads through a milk tooth far faster than through permanent teeth. Dentists will fill milk teeth in the normal manner should they need to, using exactly the same equipment as for adults, and whenever poss-ible will give a local anaesthetic (an injection) to prevent discomfort. However, they will probably use a tooth coloured *glass-ionomer* filling material, which releases fluoride into the cavity. Although too soft to fill the biting surfaces of permanent teeth it is suitable for short-life milk teeth.

Parents often worry about 'black tooth'. This occurs when a small child, often around two or three years old, falls face-first and bangs her or his upper front teeth. The tooth becomes loose, and after a time it turns grey, then almost black. Although it looks somewhat startling there is no need to be concerned unless the gum above the tooth starts to look different. This indicates an abscess, and you should consult the dentist. But if pain continues well after the fall, it might be prudent to see the dentist for x-rays to see if other damage has been done.

Extractions of milk teeth are most often done when the tooth has become decayed and an abscess has formed. They may be done with an injection. However, when a child is very unhappy, or when there is swelling, a general anaesthetic (gas) may be needed. This will probably have to be undertaken at a hospital or at a local centre that specializes in such treatments, as a diminishing number of dentists offer this service.

Both you and the dentist should keep a firm eye on that first molar tooth. If it starts to show any signs of decay in this age range then it is quite clear that the sweet intake is far too high or the cleaning pattern is all wrong or both. And this will not bode well for the rest of the permanent teeth, when they come through. It is a barometer of dental health.

Chapter Seven

Children and Young People

The eruption of the replacement permanent teeth, and the shedding of milk teeth, can occur over quite a wide time range. Furthermore, there are variations between individual children, so that the timetable below is only a guide, not a blueprint. The approximate order and timing are as follows (see in Figure 6).

- Lower incisors (1s and 2s) replace the 'a's and 'b's at 6 to 8 years.
- Upper incisors (1s and 2s) replace the 'a's and 'b's at 7 to 9 years.
- Lower canines (3s) replace the lower 'c's at 9 to 10 years.
- First premolars (4s), upper and lower, replace the 'd's at 10 to 11 years.
- Upper canines (3s) replace the upper 'c's at 11 to 12 years.
- Second premolars (5s), upper and lower, replace the 'e's at 11 to 12 years.

As a rule of thumb, the earlier the milk teeth come through the earlier they will fall out. While the loss of 'e's signal the end of the milk teeth there are still another eight permanent teeth to erupt. The second molars (the 7s) come through at around 12 years, and may actually

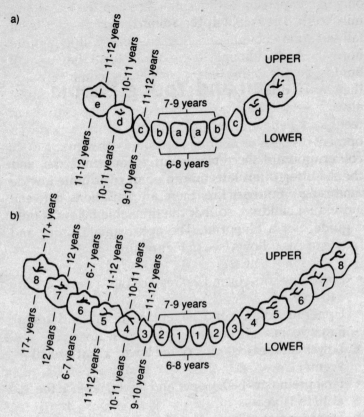

Figure 6 (a) Loss of milk teeth; (b) eruption of permanent teeth

erupt before the last milk tooth is lost. The very last molar, (the 8 or wisdom tooth) can erupt in, or after, the late teens. Together this gives the full complement of thirty-two teeth.

Children themselves, but more often parents, sometimes worry about the size, shape and colour of the front permanent teeth. But while they often look large, it is only in comparison with a small face and the remaining milk teeth. The face will grow and the other milk teeth fall out soon enough, and then the size will look quite normal. And although some front teeth have small bumps on the biting edge when they come through, they wear down very quickly. Milk teeth are almost always very white, so in comparison the permanent teeth look yellow or dull. Unless one of the rare development diseases or fluoride mottling is present the tooth colouring is almost certainly perfectly normal, and once the milk teeth fall out, and the comparison cannot be made, the problem is forgotten.

Problems with Eruption of Permanent Teeth

Sometimes one of the permanent teeth does not come through as expected. This may be because it is missing altogether (most often the upper 5s and upper 2s), other times because there is no space for it and/or it is lying in a funny position – sometimes horizontally – in the jaw bone. This tends to happen to the upper canines (3s) and the lower wisdom teeth. At other times a milk tooth does not drop out at all, and this can be quite noticeable. Often (but not always) this indicates that the relevant permanent tooth is missing.

Although there is often a considerable variation between children in the ages at which their permanent teeth come through, it is readily apparent in any one child whether one or two of the teeth are not conforming to that child's general pattern of tooth development.

These cases indicate a visit to the dentist for x-rays, which will show whether the permanent teeth are present at all, and if so whether they can be 'persuaded' to fill their proper role. If this involves the upper canine teeth, which are essential to the formation of the shape of the mouth, it is worth doing what can be quite extensive treatment using surgical techniques to expose the tooth, and orthodontic techniques to move it to its proper position. Where no tooth is present it is prudent to wait until adulthood to decide what future any retained milk teeth may have. They can be replaced with either a partial denture or a bridge.

The Dangers

Childhood is an age of acute dental danger. Appetites are at their peak and pocket money finds easily accessible sweets. Tooth decay is at its most insidious. And there are accidents with falls, balls, bats and fists impacting on the front teeth. So expensive treatment is best delayed if clinically possible. Add to this the possibility that the permanent teeth are crooked, overlapping or undershot, and that young people (especially girls) are starting to become concerned about the physical impression they make, and this becomes an age of many dental visits.

Preventive Measures

Dental necessities change with age. At the younger ages, from seven to twelve, and certainly as the permanent teeth come through, it is wise to have the crevices of the permanent back teeth sealed with a form of plastic to minimize tooth decay on the biting surface. We shall return to this preventive treatment in Chapter 13. It has to be said that this technique remains a preoccupation of dentists and parents, rather than the children themselves. And it is at these ages that broken and cracked teeth are not that uncommon, especially among boys. Although these injuries may continue among the more sporty youngsters through their teens, by then many should be wearing bite-guards to protect their teeth and jaws from various sporting impacts.

Problems with Appearance

Thumb sucking may continue until around puberty, pulling the upper teeth forward, necessitating remedial orthodontic treatment, but this does not generally preoccupy young people themselves until puberty strikes, when appearance suddenly can become everything. At this time, even an obvious fixed orthodontic appliance will be tolerated if it holds the promise of perfectly aligned teeth at a later date.

It is at this point in life that young people start to believe that they are ugly and their physical attributes not up to par. This includes the teeth. Many teenagers (by now not their parents) believe that their teeth are ugly and misshapen, even when they are not, or believe that their teeth are the wrong colour. Much effort is expended in trying to clean the teeth to a whiter-than-white, or even trying to persuade the dentist to crown them to make them shapelier or whiter. But, of course, teeth are not pure white, they are various shades of creamy colours, and white permanent teeth look very strange indeed.

Remedial Treatment

Sometimes, however, youngsters are correct about their appearance. Teeth that have been struck hard, but not broken, most often die and turn a rather sinister shade of grey. There may also be fluoride or developmental mottling, while crooked, misplaced or missing teeth and lower jaws that stick out or recede can cause acute embarrassment. But all of these can be remedied by the dentist with some of the straightforward procedures we detail in Chapter 13.

Many of these procedures involve orthodontists, but treatment is unlikely to start until the onset of puberty, at around 11 or 12. This is because the growth spurt that starts at this point aids orthodontic treatment. It is also wiser to await the arrival of all the permanent teeth, so as to be able to assess how much space will be available for tooth movements. However, if there are obvious jaw misalignments some orthodontists may wish to start treatment somewhat earlier. See Chapter 13.

Decay

Some youngsters get many more decayed teeth than others. As we have already indicated, these are probably the young people who do not clean their teeth adequately. This matters particularly if they are prone to decay. And whether they are prone to decay or not is probably a matter of luck. Different genes lead to different circumstances. One person may have a higher percentage of bacteria in the mouth, another may have less saliva, and yet another may have a tooth shape that both retains food and makes plaque deposits more difficult to clean away. There is also that positive relationship between the use of fluoride toothpaste and non-decayed teeth. Some young people use it; some do not.

Lumps

Parents may become concerned at the appearance of a small, wobbly lump, especially on a child's lower lip. It is almost certainly a *mucocele*, probably caused by a blow from a ball, or perhaps lip-biting. Although they have a habit of recurring, they are totally harmless. It is worth remembering that it is unusual in the extreme for any difficult lump to occur in the mouth until people are past their fortieth birthdays. Some teenagers become martyrs to aphthous ulcers (see Chapter 13, page 134). Regrettably there is very little they can do about them, except use a chlorhexidine mouthwash to aid healing.

Gum Disease

While the gums of young people may bleed when brushing, advanced gum disease is very rare among young people. However, it is probably starting at this time. The early signs of gum damage, and indeed loss of bone, can be detected in some teenagers, so it is important for them not only to clean their teeth thoroughly but also to go to their dentist to get good oral hygiene instructions and regular monitoring. This is the age group when not only are dental check-ups at their most important, they should also be at their most frequent.

Chapter Eight

Adults

It is a sad fact that only a minority of adults have managed to keep all their thirty-two teeth into early middle age. Decay, gum problems and accidents have taken their toll. Things could be worse, however. Today we have fillings, bridges, crowns and dentures; in Shakespeare's time most of us were 'sans teeth' by the end of adulthood. However, some things remain the same; despite these advances, today, as then, pain is associated with teeth.

Toothache

Toothache is what drives so many of us to the dentist, almost despite ourselves. It can be the worst of all possible pains, so bad as to be almost unbearable. There are times when we would happily allow a dentist to remove all our teeth if it would guarantee a good night's sleep or a good day's work. In fact, toothache has been measured to be third in intensity behind the pains of childbirth and some terminal cancers. You might think that all toothaches are the same, but in fact they are very different. We can describe a number of different types.

- Pain caused by cold air or by cold drinks and food, such as ice cream. This is likely to be caused by exposed dentine resulting from wear and tear on the teeth. Dentine that has been exposed as a result of decay or part of a tooth breaking off may be sensitive to hot food and drinks as well as cold ones.
- Pain caused by sweet drinks or sugary food. Causes as above, but more likely to be decay.
- Severe, longer-lasting pain triggered by the above two – or even coming totally out of the blue – indicates the involvement of the 'nerve' of the tooth.
- Pain caused by pressing or biting on a tooth. This is generally caused by a dead tooth having an acute *area* or abscess, or a fracture of either a filling or a tooth. Other causes of this type of pain are high (proud) fillings or crowns after a visit to the dentist. This pain can also be caused by infections around a wisdom tooth that is not fully erupted (*impacted*).
- Continual pain like a gnawing headache can be caused by severe gum problems or a tooth near to dying, with the nerve of the tooth very swollen.
- A similar pain can be caused by soft tissues, the gum or cheek. Typically this is caused by biting on the pad of gum over an impacted wisdom tooth, or an aphthous ulcer (see Chapter 13).
- Pain caused by traumatic injury. This is generally a cracked or broken tooth, although it could also be a jaw fracture.

Wisdom Teeth

Wisdom teeth are the last teeth to erupt in the mouth, from the age of 18 onwards. They are at the back of the mouth. Because all the other teeth are through, if the jaw bone is not long enough there may be no space, or insufficient space, for the wisdom teeth to occupy. This tends to be more common with the lower than with the top wisdom teeth. If you check your lower jaw you can both see and feel the jaw rise at right angles from the horizontal tooth-bearing part. This is the angle of the jaw, and it is where impacted wisdom teeth often get trapped.

An impacted wisdom tooth may be totally unerupted, in which case it rarely gives trouble. However, it may be only partially erupted, with part of the crown in the mouth. Because there is a pad of gum over the rest of the tooth, and it may well be difficult to clean adequately, the upper teeth, especially the upper wisdom teeth, bite on the gum. This leads to inflammation and infections known as *pericoronitis*. This is the main cause of wisdom tooth pain. Antibiotics are often prescribed to remove the infection.

X-rays will reveal in which of the five basic positions the partially erupted tooth may be lying. These are either vertically or horizontally or at an angle, and, if one of the latter two, the crown may be pointing towards the middle of the mouth or towards the back of the mouth. Treatment will depend on the position of the tooth. The upper wisdom teeth, generally easy to extract, are sometimes removed to avoid the pressure on the gum pad. This is done in preference to surgical extraction of the lower wisdom teeth, in which a part of a nerve can be damaged, leading to numbness of one side of the bottom lip and perhaps tongue. Because of this, oral surgeons now make patients more aware of all the possible post-operative complications.

Non-tooth 'Toothache'

There are times when 'toothaches' are not caused by teeth at all. A common cause of this patient's misdiagnosis is sinusitis. The roots of the upper teeth are very close to the lower floor of the maxillary sinus, the space inside the cheek bones that gives our voice its resonance. Sinusitis and blocked noses tend to go together. As the tooth roots are so close to the inflamed and swollen sinus, the brain misinterprets the information. The upper teeth hurt when they are clenched tightly, when putting ones foot down firmly (indeed just walking), or when lowering the head. Aphthous ulcers on the gums also can be responsible for the feeling of toothache. Neuralgia can also feel like a particularly severe toothache, especially as it is associated with the trigeminal nerve.

This nerve and its branches (one of them is involved with lower wisdom teeth), provides the sensory system for all of one side of the teeth, mouth and most of the head and face. This widespread distribution leads to another toothache problem. There are times when you are not entirely certain which tooth is hurting, indeed you may not be able to tell whether it is a top or bottom one, although you can identify the side. This is why dentists can sometimes surprise a patient by getting rid of their pain by treating a totally different tooth to the one they think is causing the trouble.

Sensitive Teeth

Some people's teeth become sensitive to hot and cold at around this age. As we explained earlier, the enamel over the crown of the tooth and the cementum covering the root are both insensitive. But on some teeth, on some people, the dentine has been exposed (see Figure 7). This might be as a result of gum disease, over-forceful brushing (*abrasion*), wear-and-tear, tooth grinding or severe erosion from gastric refluxes caused by indigestion.

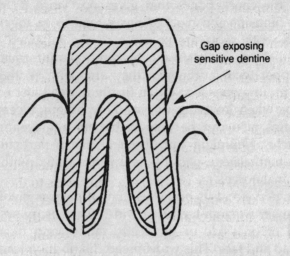

Gap exposing sensitive dentine

Figure 7 Exposed dentine due to gum disease, erosion

This condition makes a tooth (or teeth) sensitive to touch and to hot, sweet and cold substances, even cold air. It can be extremely painful. The main treatments are to reduce the acidity of the diet (especially citrus fruits) and to use a specific desensitizing toothpaste such as Sensodyne. They really do work. The dentist can also apply fluoride gel.

Gum Disease

As we have already suggested, our dental priorities – and the toothaches – change with age. We are now dealing with the age bracket where there is a crossover from rampant decay to serious gum disease. Tooth decay does not go away, but it appears to slow down. Meanwhile it is highly likely that gum disease, which has always been with us, is now apparently accelerating. However, this is misleading impression. It is not so much accelerating as accumulating (see Figure 8).

Gum disease (*periodontal disease*) is insidious. In its earlier stages it creeps along with few symptoms, and for the most part without pain.

Gum disease is caused by bacterial plaque inflaming the gums at the edge of the teeth. This leads to the most common early symptoms, glossy red (rather than stippled pink) inflamed and bleeding gums. If the plaque is not cleaned away, saliva – which contains salts – calcifies it to create calculus. This is why calculus is laid down most heavily on the inside of the lower teeth and the outside of the upper back teeth, where the salivary glands are sited. Calculus is hard and rough and attracts even more plaque. This irritates the gum even further, creating more swelling and bleeding. The plaque causes a breakdown of the fibres holding the tooth to the bone, creating a *gingival pocket* between the root of the tooth and the gum. Some of the bone supporting the teeth is lost as the pocket forms. Plaque then starts to calcify to form calculus in the pocket beneath the gum level. More plaque is laid down, and more fibres which secure the tooth to the bone then start to break down, and more bone is lost, deepening the pocket. In turn this leaves

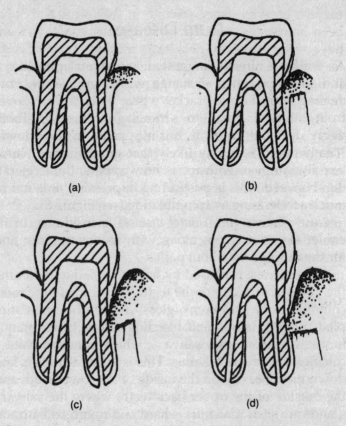

Figure 8 Progression of gum disease: (a) plaque inflames the gums at the edge of the teeth and forms calculus; (b) fibres holding the tooth to the bone break down, forming a gingival pocket, and some of the supporting bone is lost; (c) and (d) calculus forms in the pocket, more fibres break down, more bone is lost, and the pocket deepens

more space for food to get trapped and plaque and calculus to get deposited, so deepening the pocket even further. A vicious circle has been created.

This usually happens over decades, rather than

months or even years, starting in the teens. If this has been happening, and the gum remains intact, you will have deep gingival pocketing around most of your teeth. However, the danger is that looking in the mirror it might appear that all is well as your gums are at their normal level.

As fibres and bone are lost the tooth progressively becomes looser, until it becomes impossible to retain. The process is irreversible, although treatment at an early enough stage can halt the process, but only if it is associated with improved oral hygiene. Prevention is not just far better than cure, it is essential, and good plaque removal at all ages, especially in this period of life when all might seem well, is vital for the halting of this disease.

Gumboils

The 'pockets' around the teeth are also prone to infections that can cause acute gumboils (*periodontal abscesses*, see Figure 9a). In essence these are no different from any other abscess, a result of the body defending itself against an infection. They are full of pus, which is just a collection of dead tissue and white blood cells that have died in the cause of stopping the infection spreading. There are also chronic infections where pus drains persistently into the mouth through the gap between the tooth and the bone. This results in both a bad taste and bad breath smells. Both infections destroy the supporting bone.

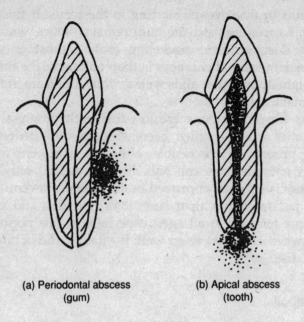

(a) Periodontal abscess
(gum)

(b) Apical abscess
(tooth)

Figure 9

A second form of gumboil is a tooth abscess caused by a tooth dying, perhaps the result of a blow or decay reaching the *pulp* (the 'nerve'). This is called an *apical abscess* (see Figure 9b). The process leading to the tooth dying may be extremely painful, although at other times it may not be noticed at all. Pain is caused by an acute inflammation or infection of the pulp. This is soft tissue with both a blood and nerve supply. The infection and inflammation make it swell up. But as there is nowhere for this swelling to expand, the pulp effectively strangles itself. This increased pressure adds its own characteristic dimension to the pain. As the pulp is the only conductor of blood (and so oxygen) to the tooth, once the pulp has died, the tooth has also died.

The infection in the pulp tracks to the end of the tooth (the *apex*) and into the bone. It can either bide its time here quietly, or it can almost explode. In the former case it tends to create what is known as an *area*, after its x-ray appearance, a dark area in lighter bone. It may also form a cyst, which is a space filled with fluid contained in a membrane. In the acute version, the infection (the abscess) cannot escape through the tooth into the mouth, so it tracks through the bone along the lines of the weakest parts. This causes typical swelling. Pain also occurs when pressure is put on the tooth. Only when the pus reaches the outside through the gum and discharges into the mouth is the pain relieved. For treatments see Chapter 13.

Restorative Techniques

This is the age where teeth that have already been filled need larger fillings or crowns, or get so decayed they have to be extracted. It follows that it is also the age of bridge work and partial dentures. Bridges, like bridges in the wider world, span a gap. They are basically false teeth attached permanently to other teeth. While partial dentures also replace one or more missing teeth, they are, like all dentures, removable. We shall go into more detail about restorative dental techniques in Chapters 9 and 13.

Erosion, Attrition and Abrasion

One particularly specific problem is the erosion of teeth that comes from regurgitating food and stomach contents. This is a particular problem with people suffering from bulimia and anorexia. A typical characteristic of bulimics, who binge after a period of anorexic non-eating and then force themselves to vomit, is that the backs of their front teeth are dissolved by their acid regurgitations. This problem is also common among that large percentage of the population who suffer regularly from various forms of indigestion, and who typically buy and munch antacid tablets. The stomach's hydrochloric acid can eat teeth away with surprising ease and to a surprising degree. The erosion can be seen on all tooth surfaces, especially the inside of both upper and lower teeth. It can also start surprisingly early in life. A 1993 government-sponsored dental health survey showed tooth erosion was significant among teenagers, especially those with diets heavy in sugar and carbonated drinks.

The same degree of enamel loss and wear can come from tooth grinding (*bruxism*), although generally this affects the biting surfaces of teeth, not their front and inside surfaces. This is known as *attrition*. Teeth can also suffer from *abrasion*. This is caused by an outside agent physically rubbing against the teeth. Typically it will be over-enthusiastic brushing, especially with a very hard brush, and/or using abrasive toothpastes or toothpaste substitutes. Some smokers' toothpastes are very abrasive. Abrasion can affect all tooth surfaces, but especially the outer (lip) surface where the tooth meets the gum.

Nowadays we rarely need to chew vigorously, indeed the quality of food is often judged by its tenderness rather than its flavour. This means we tend to add spices, sugars and acid-based flavourings, all of which add to dental decay formation. Short of going back to pre-industrial diets and eating foodstuffs that contain little sugar, require steady chewing and tearing, and do not just adhere to the teeth, all we can do is take preventive and remedial actions.

Pregnancy

Old wives' tales still abound in this sphere of life. For example, it is not true that calcium is taken from a pregnant woman's teeth to add calcium to the baby's bones and teeth. Nor is it true that a pregnant woman should expect to lose at least one tooth for every baby. It *is* true that exaggerated responses to hormonal levels may create soft, spongy gums that bleed at the slightest touch, and occasionally create small spongy growths of gum tissue (*pyogenic granulomas*). However, after pregnancy the gums will resume their normal colour, state and health. And apart from this, there is no reason why teeth and gums should deteriorate in pregnancy.

When tooth and mouth trouble does occur during pregnancy, it is generally caused by poor oral hygiene, which is largely due to preoccupations with other matters. But if the following advice is observed, teeth and gums can remain healthy throughout pregnancy.

- Maintain a healthy, balanced diet. This is important for the development of the baby's teeth and bones.
- Take far greater care to clean teeth and maintain oral hygiene than when not pregnant.
- Use a chlorhexidine mouthwash.
- If morning sickness makes teeth cleaning difficult, change the schedule and clean teeth before bedtime.
- While most dental treatments are perfectly safe during pregnancy, bleeding, swollen gums make it inadvisable to prepare crowns and bridges. These should be left until after birth.

Even if all appears well, pregnant women should visit their dentist in the first couple of months to discuss any possible problems, and again towards the end of pregnancy to check on what has been happening to the gums and teeth. As NHS dentistry is free during pregnancy and for a year afterwards, it is also financially advantageous to take advantage of this and get needed treatment done. X-rays are not normally taken in pregnancy, although the latest research suggests they do no harm.

Chapter Nine

The Older Mouth

Care of the mouth and teeth at this age is more important than ever, despite the fact that few elderly people have all or even most of their teeth. For the most part people in their sixties, and certainly into their seventies, have dentures, or other replacement teeth of some description.

Older Teeth

As you get older it is vital to maintain your oral hygiene, even if you have lost some or perhaps most of your teeth. This is because increasing age, some medications (for high blood pressure for example) and radiotherapy all decrease saliva flows, and as we have seen this hinders acid neutralization on the teeth. Taken together with an increased consumption of sweet hot drinks, biscuits between meals and sweets (mints and cough sweets are a feature of the diets of elderly people), these can all lead to a veritable explosion of tooth decay. Very careful and thorough removal of plaque is vital. Regular rinsing with a fluoride mouthwash at bedtime will also help keep decay at bay.

There are additional tooth problems at this older age. Over time, teeth wear down on their biting edges.

Typically the enamel wears away on the biting surface and the dentine is exposed. As the exposed dentine is softer than enamel it wears away more quickly, leaving unsupported ledges of enamel which then break off. Once this condition has started it accelerates rapidly. This leaves the teeth with very short crowns, which are both unsightly and inefficient at biting. The exposed dentine also may be very painful. It is both complicated and expensive to remedy this condition.

A variant is the loss of enamel at the level of the gum. At this time of life the gum may well be receding, showing a considerable portion of the root of the tooth. This gives rise to the description of a person as 'long in the tooth'. The exposed dentine is not only painful, all too often it also becomes a collar of rampant decay around the root surface, as people find it painful to clean the plaque away from this area. Specialist desensitizing toothpastes must be used, especially as it is very difficult for the dentist to fill these cavities successfully. A new treatment is becoming available, which seals this decay and to some extent reverses the process (see Chapter 14).

Bridges and Dentures

If your mouth is shared between your own teeth and perhaps a partial denture and/or bridge(s), maintaining your oral hygiene takes on an additional financial incentive. It is important to keep the remaining teeth for as long as possible. Not only are your own teeth better at biting and chewing, but the remaining teeth may be vital to the stability and retention of an existing denture, and certainly a bridge. There may even be metal clasps of a partial denture around some of your own teeth. Although it is possible to add teeth to a denture, the entire denture may have to be redesigned and remade. This can be both expensive and time-consuming. The same applies to a tooth to which a bridge is attached. Once that has been lost, the bridge is also lost. So it is more efficient, cheaper and easier to ensure that the teeth next to the denture, or those that support bridges, are pristine. They must be kept plaque-free.

Both full and partial dentures may well be 'immediate' dentures. That is to say that the denture has been made before the teeth are extracted, and fitted immediately after extraction, at the same appointment. Within six months, the part of the gum where the extraction took place, which is now in contact with the fitting surface of the denture, will have 'shrunk'. The denture starts to feel loose, rather like a dress or pair of trousers after a bout of slimming. This is called *bone resorption* and is perfectly natural. It generally means that either the denture will have to be re-based or you will need a new one. Resorption is a more difficult problem with full dentures, as the poor fit becomes far more noticeable. At one time people who needed full dentures were made to wait for almost six months while the bone 'shrank' before a dentist would make them. Today, immediate dentures are more common.

There are various types of dentures and other tooth replacements. Although we shall cover them more thoroughly in Chapter 13, it is worthwhile outlining the salient points.

- All dentures are removable.
- They either replace some teeth (partial) or all the

83

teeth (full).
- They can be made of plastic or metal (generally cast chrome-cobalt steel).
- The upper ones can cover the entire roof of the mouth, or be in 'skeleton' form.
- The teeth are usually made of plastic.

Dentures are never as good as your own teeth. In particular, full upper and lower dentures can be difficult to keep stable. This can make eating difficult. Partial dentures fill gaps between teeth. Because of this, and unlike full dentures, they vary widely in type and construction. There may be as many as three or four different sections of false teeth on the plate, separated by the natural teeth, or it may be a single tooth replacement. There are also metal partial skeleton dentures, which cover less gum and roof of the mouth, but have metal arms extending around the cheek surfaces of the back teeth. Other partial dentures have clasps onto teeth, and may be extremely small.

Dentures are made to fit each individual mouth. Lower full dentures sit on a narrow ridge and can be difficult to control; upper dentures are more stable as they have suction imparted by the hard palate. Some people cope with their dentures from day one, but others never come to terms with them. The difference is often psychological rather than physical or mechanical, although controlling the tongue in order to stop it dislodging the lower denture requires perseverance.

While appearance is important, you have to eat with dentures, not just look as though you have all your own teeth. Denture fixative is used by many people, but only works on the upper denture. So most people with full dentures have to learn to adapt their diet. Apples and other hard foods may need to be pre-cut or sliced. Chewy meats are likely to be forsworn, as are foods with small pips, which can find their way under dentures and cause irritation.

Dentures should be removed from the mouth and cleaned daily. Cleaning is in two parts. All dentures should be scrubbed carefully with a hard brush, reaching into all the nooks and crannies to remove plaque. They should also be cleaned by a soaking in a commercial denture cleanser, although it is not necessary to leave your dentures to soak overnight. Never use bleach or other self-selected cleaning agents as these tend to damage the plastic. Very small dentures should be removed at night – or when playing energetic sports – as they can get dislodged and obstruct the airway.

The gums on which dentures rest also have to be kept in good condition, and this includes brushing the roof of your mouth and gums with a toothbrush and toothpaste. Sore spots or ulcers should be treated speedily, especially if they follow the fitting of new dentures. However, the denture may well need 'easing' by the dentist, and a chlorhexidine mouthwash or gel is useful in helping the gums recover. This also applies to aphthous ulcers. It is also possible for the root of a long-forgotten tooth, which has been buried in the bone painlessly for many years, to work its way to the surface of the mouth. This will cause pain under a denture and it should be removed by the dentist. Some people never come to terms with their dentures, especially full sets. In such cases, other forms of replacement might be indicated, such as implants.

Lumps and Bumps

If a lump, bump or ulcer appears in the mouth and does not disappear within a fortnight, go to the dentist. While tumours in the mouth are rare they do occur. Most are relatively harmless, a few others are not. As most of the invasive tumours appear later in life, this advice is more pertinent to the older person. This advice includes the sides of the tongue and salivary glands, which can be found on the sides of either cheek and on either side beneath the tongue. There is also the possibility that the duct of the salivary gland can become blocked with a little stone, creating pain until it is removed.

Advancing age not only affects the mouth and teeth, it affects the body and mind. This may result in an inability to undertake teeth cleaning or other maintenance of teeth or dentures. But it is important that these are done by carers, and that treatment by the dentist, if required, is not curtailed by handicaps. Home visits by the dentist may be vital. In some instances this has to be the responsibility of the carer, as the decision-making ability of the person may be severely impaired.

And one thing must be remembered. It doesn't matter if you are nineteen or ninety – if you need a crown or a bridge then have it made. Age should be no barrier to having and maintaining a healthy mouth and teeth. So at the very least, if manual dexterity or eyesight is becoming impaired, make an appointment with your dentist to discuss what the best ways of managing your mouth might be.

Part Three

At the Dentist

Chapter Ten

The People

When you go to a typical dental practice you will meet
not only the dentist but also various other people. This
chapter explains who they are and what they do. We
shall also explain the many varieties of dentists, some
of whom you may come across in hospitals, in dental
schools and in non-NHS speciality practices.

Dentists

Surgeons in Britain drop the title doctor. All dentists
are dental surgeons. This explains why medical surgeons
and dentists are called Mr, Miss, Mrs or Ms, rather than
Dr, as in the USA and the rest of the European Union. As
of November 1995, however, dentists can use the title
doctor if they wish. The two basic qualifications you will
come across most often on the brass plate, letterheads or
business cards of general practice dentists are:

- Bachelor of Dental Surgery (BDS), followed by the
  University where the dentist trained, e.g. (London),
  (Manchester) or perhaps (Sydney).
- Licentiate in Dental Surgery, Royal College of
  Surgeons (LDS RCS).

Most dentists go on refresher courses and attend seminars to learn about the latest techniques. Some of these are part of their NHS conditions of service, especially for the older dentists; others are done in their own time and at their own expense. Many specialists visit the USA regularly for this purpose.

Since the single market, the EU has insisted that all registered practitioners are allowed to cross borders to practise. However, it appears that in some countries scant regard is paid to proper qualifications – except in theory. A specialist orthodontist practising in an EU capital city provides an example. He boasts of his degree – an unusual occurrence for an orthodontist in his city. However, it is a law degree; he has no dental qualifications at all, but can earn more money as an orthodontist than as a lawyer. The same regulations are also diluting UK specialities, and there are fears at the highest levels that standards could fall. Until this matter has been resolved (and work on it is in hand at the moment; see Chapter 14, we can only urge you to be cautious should you be faced with a dentist with an EU-registered qualification other than UK or Irish. While most will be professionally competent, some will not.

You may see other basic dental degrees (BDSc and BChD) and many non-specific dental post-graduate degrees. These include Masters (MDS); Doctorate (PhD), and Fellowship (FDS RCS). In addition to these there are qualifications in general dental practice and community dentistry, but these are more about professional careers than of concern to patients.

Specializations

While at present it is not lawful for dental surgeons to describe themselves as 'specialists', there is an increasing number of dental surgeons who have obtained extra qualifications in their chosen specialities. Many of these have a Masters (MSc) degree, or perhaps a PhD, that is specific to their area of expertise. This generally means a minimum of a two-year course involving both theory and additional practical skills. Among these specialists are:

- **Prosthetists**. These are dentists who specialize in the designing, making and fitting of dentures. Although there are some in private practice, the majority are in dental hospitals.
- **Periodontists**. These are dentists who specialize in diagnosing, controlling and treating gum diseases. While there are a few in private practice, most are found in dental hospitals.
- **Oral surgeons**. These are dentists who specialize in surgery in and around the mouth. Some are also medically qualified. Their case load can range over the removal of wisdom teeth, implants and the removal of small tumours and plastic surgery. They are found mainly in general and dental hospitals.
- **Conservationists**. These are dentists whose job is to preserve teeth by using advanced techniques, such as crown and bridge work, implants and full mouth rehabilitation. Many are found in private practice and in dental hospitals.
- **Endodontists**. These are dentists who specialize in saving teeth by root-treating them. There are very

few of them in UK private practice and dental hospitals.

- **Orthodontists**. These are dentists who specialize in straightening teeth. Their areas of expertise, however, can go far further than this. They also have their own diploma (Dip Orth) which is a step on the road to even higher degrees. They are found in specialist NHS and private practices, as well as both dental and large general hospitals.
- **Oral pathologists**. These are dentists who specialize in oral and maxillo-facial diseases. They diagnose and manage the treatment of the mouth tissues, bones and the salivary glands.

It is important to realize that by and large you will have to be referred to one of the above by your own dentist. Then, one of two things will happen. Either you will be treated by the expert, or the expert will provide a treatment plan for your own dentist. Which route is chosen depends on the problem, what your dentist asked for, and the facilities and expertise available at your own dentist.

Other Key People

Apart from the dentist, you may come across a number of people at the dental surgery, with various skills and expertise:

- **Receptionist/practice manager**. The first person you will meet or talk to at the dental surgery is the receptionist. Given that first impressions are important, an efficient receptionist and/or practice manager is priceless to the dental practice. With the increasing size of dental practices and vastly increased NHS paperwork and bureaucracy, there is an increasing need for practice managers, especially those skilled in the use of computers.

- **Dental nurse**. Also known as a dental surgery assistant, the dental nurse is vital to any surgery, and can comfort a nervous patient and ease the burden on the dentist. Sometimes the dental nurse needs to be psychic, and have instruments or materials ready before being asked for them. They can be formally trained and get National Vocational Qualifications in courses run under the auspices of BTec.

- **Dental ancillary**. Also known as 'dental therapists', dental ancillaries must work under the direction of a qualified dentist. They perform simple fillings, extractions of milk teeth with simple local anaesthetic, sealing techniques and oral hygiene matters on children in the community dental service. They undertake a one-year training course leading to a qualification.

- **Dental hygienist**. There are many dental hygienists working in general practice, often on a part-time basis, dividing their time between surgeries. They work under the supervision of dentists on scalings and oral hygiene instruction. They can also be found in practices specializing in gum diseases to which patients must be referred by general dental practitioners. They undertake a one-year training course leading to a qualification.

- **Dental technician**. Dental technicians work in a dental laboratory making dentures, crowns, bridges and orthodontic appliances, although they will specialize in only one of these. They are not often seen by patients, even when they are working on the surgery premises, but you may meet a technician (ceramicist) when colour matching a private crown, bridge or denture.

There are also **denturists**. Although actually illegal in the UK, they do exist. Basically they are dental technicians who specialize in the manufacture and repair of dentures, but who will also undertake to make dentures from the first visit to the final article. They operate from shops, laboratories and from home. They do not work from dental surgeries, nor will they be seen in them. If detected they are prosecuted.

Chapter Eleven

The Equipment

Not that many years ago, certainly post–1945, some dental surgeries were still equipped with treadle-operated drills (like old-fashioned sewing machines), and patients sat almost bolt upright with the dentist standing while she or he worked. Nowadays we are in the era of air-turbine drills, ultrasonic scalers and patients lying almost horizontal. Clearly there have been startling advances in dental techniques and in the type and standard of equipment used since those days.

Surgery Design

Yet there can also be startling differences in the way today's dental surgeries are both arranged and equipped. This is not only a matter of the age or design of equipment, it also reflects both the physical requirements of individual dentists and their approach to patients. These differences are manifested in what a dentist wears. Some wear white or blue smocks or coats; others work in ordinary clothes. Some dentists habitually wear a face-mask; others rarely wear one. And while most dentists now wear surgical gloves and protective spectacles, some still do not. In smaller practices, the dentist imposes his or her personality on the surgery design; in group or branch practices, the design is imposed on the dentist.

Dental surgeries can be in a wide variety of premises. One might be in a residential street; another in a well-known medical and dental area such as Harley Street. Others may be in purpose-built clinics, in lock-up shops or above commercial premises in the local high street. The building might be shared with doctors or other medical workers forming an unofficial medical centre, or indeed be in a new medical complex. Dental technicians may share the premises. It may be a single or multiple surgery practice. Some surgeries and waiting rooms are light and airy; others small and windowless.

While some surgeries are designed so that the equipment is hidden in recesses or cupboards until it is required, others are dominated by large chunks of surgery furniture. But whatever the style, all dental surgeries need somewhere for the patient to sit, a good light source and a module with instruments and facilities that both the dentist and you, the patient, can reach without undue stretching. Despite the large number of available variations, these are the essentials without which dentists cannot operate successfully. This chapter will outline and explain what you see when you get into a dental surgery, and what everything is used for.

The Essentials

The following are the main features of a typical dental surgery.

The chair

The modern dental chair is a work of science fiction art, in which the patient reclines rather than sits. While designs vary, all modern dental chairs move horizontally and vertically at the merest touch of a button. This allows the dentist to sit while working, and provides a good view of, and access to, the mouth. It also prevents a patient having a fainting fit.

The light

Dental lights used to look as though they had been borrowed from the Eddystone Lighthouse. Today's are smaller, with cool light focused where it is needed, not scattered around the surgery. The light can be free-hanging or it may be an integral part of the working console.

The working controls

The working controls are also called the **module** or **console**. The design of the module varies more than anything else in the dental surgery. Some are fixed entirely, some are part fixed and part mobile and others are almost entirely mobile or retractable. Part of the console is patient-oriented; most is dentist-friendly. The part you will use is the spittoon (small round sink) or funnel and the mouthwash cup; this may refill itself automatically. The dentist's part is always free-moving. It provides a working surface on which instruments and materials are placed, and a module in which the mechanical instruments (drills, air and water jets) are sited. Here they are described in more detail:

- **Drills/handpieces**. The visible part of a dentist's drill is now a metal handpiece. This is usually a complex air-turbine that holds the drill. It is driven by an air-compressor. Cutting is done by drills *(burrs)*. These are generally made of stainless steel or industrial diamond. There are different burrs for different dental jobs. The handpiece can also hold tooth-polishing equipment, and a variety of other specialist cutters and drills. It also may be equipped with a fibre-optic light. The handpiece runs at variable speeds, up to very high speeds, and so the tooth on which it is working has to be cooled by a constant jet of water running from the handpiece itself. There will also be a slower running handpiece, possibly powered by a microelectric motor.
- **Saliva ejector**. As it is not always possible to swallow easily, to avoid flooding in the mouth from the jet of water the dentist generally asks you to hold a question-mark-shaped gadget in your mouth. This is a suction-based saliva ejector, and it sucks up the water and your own saliva. (Alternatively, in what is called 'four-handed dentistry', the dental nurse holds the saliva ejector in place.)
- **Water and air jets**. The water jet is used to clean debris away from the tooth or gum where the dentist is working. The air-jet is then used for drying that part of the mouth. Both are very powerful, and are powered

by same air-compressor that powers the drill.
- **Electronic scaler**. This has replaced the older hand-scalers (see below) as the main method of removing gross calculus from around the teeth. It works using ultrasonics. The head of the handpiece, which contains a sickle-shaped 'scaler', runs off the central console and is powered from the central unit.

X-ray machine

In contrast to the large, forbidding x-ray machines of some fifteen years ago, when the dentist either hid in a corner or retired to another room every time an x-ray was taken, modern machines are small and have extremely low levels of stray radiation. Because they have high voltage combined with low amperage, the dose of x-rays is very low. The net effect is that patients are exposed to very little more radiation than they would get from a luminous watch. Along with many other safety aspects of the surgery, x-ray machines are monitored by a government agency (National Radiation Board). They may be free-standing (mobile) or part of the main console.

X-ray developer

This is a small machine that develops x-rays in 5 minutes. This allows a full diagnosis to be made at the primary examination stage.

Sterilizer

Sterilization is an essential part of today's dental surgery practice. There are many types available, but the one that appears to give the most comprehensive sterilization uses a combination of heat and pressure, and is called an *autoclave*. It looks like a windowless microwave oven. All non-disposable instruments are sterilized after each time of use. Antiseptic and ultrasonic bath sterilization may also be used alongside this method.

There is a monologue, 'At the Dentist' by the American comedian Shelley Berman, which starts: 'The dentist walks over to one of his cabinets, takes out a drawer, and empties it into your mouth. Then he goes away – for ever.' The contents of that drawer, and many others around the surgery, are smaller instruments – most of which have specific uses – and a large variety of materials. Here are the most common ones that you may come across:

- **Probes** are steel instruments that have a right angle at the business end, and are used both in check-ups and treatment. They can be fine-pointed for discovering decay or blunt-ended and calibrated for discovering and measuring 'pocket' depth.
- **Mouth mirrors** are used constantly by dentists. They use the light from the lamp to get a clear view of the inside of the mouth and the upper teeth.
- **Syringes** are used for giving local anaesthetics. The anaesthetic (lignocaine), which is in cartridge form (like ink for a fountain pen), and the needles are never used for more than one patient.
- **Forceps** are used for extracting teeth. They come in many shapes and sizes, with both different grips and different 'jaws' – the end that grips the tooth. Many of them are based on old designs. Each pair of forceps is used to extract specific teeth, in specific

parts of the mouth. Dentists tend to use the ones to which they have become accustomed.

- **Excavators** are small steel instruments with sharp, differently shaped ends, used for removing decay from cavities where great care is needed.
- **Elevators** are small steel instruments of different shapes that are used in the extraction of teeth, especially roots. They either work as wedges or by applying leverage.
- **Scalpels** are exactly the same as those found in operating theatres. They are used in surgical extractions, apicetomies (see page 115), or possibly gum treatments.
- **Scalers** are small metal instruments with different shaped heads: some spoon-shaped, some straight and some at right angles to the shaft, all with a sharp edge. They remove calculus from around and between the teeth and beneath the gum level. Despite the widespread use of ultrasonic scaling, they are used both to finish a scaling and to 'fine-scale' teeth when chronic gum disease demands a very close scaling.
- **Reamers** (also called files) are fine metal rods 21–28mm long and of varying widths, with a file-like exterior. They are used to clear out and widen the root canals of teeth prior to their being root-filled.
- **Impression trays** are carriers of impression material. Upper trays look like a shovel with a large part for the roof of the mouth. Lower trays have a horseshoe shape. The impressions are used by technicians to create plaster models of the upper and lower jaws. These are then used to make dentures, orthodontic appliances, bite guards, crowns, bridges and other dental appliances.

- **Pluggers and carvers** are small metal instruments. The former (which have a ball at one end and a tiny hammerhead at the other) are used to compress amalgam into cavities, the latter are used to make the filling tooth-shaped.
- **Matrix bands and holders** are used in combination: the bands are inserted around the teeth and tightened into position using the holder. They form an artificial tooth wall when one has been removed in the cutting of a cavity. The filling material is packed into this bounded space. Without this wall on this sort of filling, the filling material would be packed onto the gum between the teeth, giving a weak, ill fitting filling, and subsequent gum problems.
- **Rubber dam**. Used by some dentists to isolate a tooth, keeping it moisture free. Some patients find the rubber (which is clamped around the tooth and stretched tautly) extremely unpleasant. Others, including habitual 'gaggers', can find it a much more pleasant experience.
- **Shade guides**. Collections of plastic incisor teeth used to match or determine the colour of dentures and crowns.
- **Polymerization light**. This is an intensified light source (often blue but not ultra-violet) used to harden plastic filling materials in the mouth when fissure sealing, filling a tooth, or lining a cavity.

There are also many things you will not see. The clinical waste bin and 'sharps box' isolate possibly contaminated garbage. And the electrics and plumbing in the average dental surgery must be both state-of-the-art and reliable. There are also ultrasonic bath sterilizers, warm-air driers and both an air-compressor and electric motor housing.

The most common disposable materials you will come across, other than cotton-wool rolls and mouth-wash, are amalgam filling material and a variety of tooth-coloured filling materials (see Chapter 12). You will also discover a variety of impression materials. Some of these are used to make the impressions for dentures or bite guards. Others are capable of register-ing much finer detail and are used for bridge and crown work. The former are alginate based, derived from seaweeds. Crowns and bridges are made using impression materials based on rubber, polyvinyl or hydrocolloid.

Chapter Twelve

Filling Materials
– the Controversy

For over a hundred years the basic filling material for back teeth has been 'amalgam'. It is a mixture of mercury and a powder of silver, zinc, tin and copper. Amalgam starts soft and very pliable, can be carved into toothlike contours, but sets firm within ten minutes and hard within an hour. On the other hand, the basic front teeth filling materials, or for the front surface of all teeth, have been tooth-coloured for many years. They are made of silicate, plastic or a composite of the two.

Given that even beautifully carved and polished amalgam fillings appear black, why not use tooth-coloured filling materials? One problem is that they are difficult to manipulate satisfactorily in back teeth, and the fillings in these teeth can take very much longer than the only alternative, amalgam. But the main reason is that they wear out too quickly – and can cause fractures of back teeth. The average life of a composite filling is five years. Research shows that an average tooth can only be filled and refilled five times before it is beyond refilling. So the use of composite fillings would shorten the life of a tooth from life to twenty-five years. However, composite fillings (plastic and silicate) can be used for single surface fillings in the back teeth biting surface and milk teeth fillings.

But the problem with amalgam is not only aesthetic. It is the mercury content. Mercury has been known to be a poison for many years. Hatters used to use it to weight the brims of their hats so that they sat upright. After a lifetime of handling it, many hatters appeared to exhibit signs of mental instability, hence the description, 'mad as a hatter'. If you look closely you will see that in the dental surgery amalgam is now mixed automatically in an airtight capsule. (This is for the protection of dentists and dental nurses who otherwise would be exposed to mercury fumes.) Clearly it is a hazardous substance.

A recent BBC television programme suggested that amalgam fillings were responsible for a variety of illnesses, citing mercury as the villain of the piece. Strangely enough, although it created some concern, the reaction among patients in dental surgeries throughout the country was not as strong as might have been anticipated. Perhaps this is because most people have amalgam fillings, yet very few have experienced the problems that the programme highlighted, and those who have experienced such problems have generally found them to be caused by other factors.

While not wishing to defend amalgam entirely, the programme should not escape serious criticism. It took a series of theories and half-truths and built a logical case from them as though they were incontrovertible facts. It is rather like building your house on quicksand. If mixed properly, amalgam contains no free mercury; it all combines with the silver-based powder so that none of it is available to leak into the mouth. In August 1995, the Fédération Dentaire Internationale (FDI), the international dental organization, cooperating with the World Health Organization (WHO) issued the following statement on amalgam fillings.

Components in dental restorative materials, including amalgam, may, in rare instances, result in local side-effects or allergic reactions. A small amount of mercury is released from amalgam restorations, especially during placement and removal. However, many sources contribute to the mercury burden of individuals, including food (especially fish), water and air pollution. The risk of adverse side effects is very low for all types of restorative materials including amalgam and resin based materials. Because of the fear of possible adverse effects of mercury, some patients with a variety of symptoms may request removal of amalgam restorations. However, there is no support in the scientific literature indicating that general symptoms may be relieved by the replacement of the restorations.

There are also two distinctly different health factors in mercury use that must not be confused. The first is its toxicity. This is what the BBC programme was about. However, much of current concern about the effects of mercury, especially in Scandinavia, does not involve amalgam fillings in the mouth, which once they have hardened should not be able to release mercury. It is based on general environmental factors such as the disposal of old amalgam into public water systems and air-borne mercury vapour from crematoria. The second factor, which was referred to in the FDI/WHO statement, is that a small number of people are allergic to mercury. Clearly they cannot have amalgam fillings without being in considerable distress, even danger. But for the overwhelming majority of people this is not the case. If you believe that you might be allergic to mercury or one of the other constituents of amalgam, your doctor will arrange for the appropriate clinical tests.

In any event, however, amalgam is not the absolutely ideal filling material. Certainly it contracts and expands at the same rate as a tooth when it gets hot and cold. This is important, because it prevents a gap developing between the tooth and the filling, or the filling material expanding overmuch and shattering the tooth. But it can fracture when used for very large fillings. In such cases the only alternative is a cast crown or inlay (see Chapter 13, page 116), both of which are cemented onto the preparation. Fine-leaf gold can also be compressed and used as a filling material. The problem here is that, at present, gold-work of all descriptions is expensive.

The problem will almost certainly be extinguished in time. The current concern about mercury has increased the resources being put into dental materials research. Even now the only fillings that need to be done in amalgam are multi-surface ones on the back teeth. At this point is must be mentioned that the NHS will not pay for composite fillings in back teeth, unless a doctor certifies they are necessary for medical reasons. So tooth-coloured fillings in back teeth will need to be on a private basis. Given the time they take to do properly, and their propensity to wear out, this will be an expensive option.

Academics believe that amalgam will be phased out by the end of the century as new, tooth-coloured filling materials that fulfil all the criteria of amalgam, but with a higher tensile strength, come on stream. Until then, unless you are allergic to mercury or one of the other components of the alloy, there is no need to replace amalgam fillings. To do so would put teeth at unnecessary risk unless expensive inlay or crown conservation techniques are used.

Chapter Thirteen

The Different Treatments

In this chapter we outline the main treatments available at the dentist – in general practice, in specialist practices and in hospital clinics. While not comprehensive it will cover almost everything you are likely to come across at the dentist.

But before outlining what can be done, we must make an important overall point. Dental treatment has changed in emphasis in more recent years. Proper treatment planning has become pivotal. Dentists now manage patient's problems, as well as treat them. In other words the patient comes first, the mouth second, and the treatment third.

As a result, dentistry has become less interventionist. Partly this is because it is now realized that small decaying spots in the enamel may repair themselves in the absence of plaque and especially with fluoride applications or environment. So they can be left and watched. Partly it is because the role of plaque in tooth and gum disease was only realized in the late 1970s and only then could real preventive measures be taken. And it is also because techniques have changed. As we shall see below, changes in cavity preparation mean smaller holes; operations on the gum (gingivectomies) are rare, and apicectomies (see below, page 115) are performed less often.

We covered the examination and treatment plan in Chapter 2. The following list of treatments (and elements of treatment) is not in any order of importance, although we start with the saving of teeth.

Sealing

Sealing is an attempt to prevent decay occurring in a tooth by covering the 'fissures' on the biting surface of the permanent back teeth of young people. The tooth surface is roughed with acid (*etched*), a composite plastic is placed on the tooth surface and intensified light hardens it.

X-rays

Routine x-rays (*bite-wings*) are taken at your first visit and as necessary (depending on the state of your mouth) subsequently. Today's x-rays give a very low dose of radiation. The bite-wing is a small, rigid frame clenched between the back teeth, which holds the x-ray film at right angles to the teeth. It gives a side view of the teeth and bone. This enables the dentist to see how much bone has been lost around teeth, and whether there is decay on the tooth surfaces between the teeth. Decay shows up as darker patches in the enamel and dentine. It also shows how deep the decay goes, and whether it is likely to involve the pulp (the 'nerve'). Whole-tooth and other x-rays show abscesses, cysts or areas at the end of the root; buried roots, and unerupted or partly erupted teeth – wisdom teeth in particular. Most of these x-rays are taken on small films that you hold in position. Pan-oral x-rays show the whole mouth, laid out in one flat x-ray, and are used in orthodontic or oral surgery treatment.

Injections and Other Pain Relief

Despite widespread apprehension, there is no need to feel pain at the dentist. Any procedure likely to cause pain – extractions, fillings, etc., or even deep scalings – can be dealt with by some form of anaesthetic. Here are the main ones:

- **Local anaesthetics**, such as lignocaine, are given by injection, either in the gum above/below the tooth or by a 'block' at the back of the lower jaw. With added adrenaline (standard mixture) the numbness lasts for 2 to 3 hours; without adrenaline it lasts for about 30 minutes.
- A **general anaesthetic** is given to very nervous patients, children, for complicated procedures or when a large amount of work has to be done at a single visit. Most often done in 'gas' sessions in specialist surgeries with the anaesthetic administered by an experienced medical anaesthetist, and treatment by a dental practitioner.
- **Relative anaesthesia** is a mixture of nitrous oxide and oxygen, administered through a nosepiece. The patient is never unconscious. Although it is a very powerful analgesic (painkiller), local anaesthetics are often given as well. The technique is very similar to

the 50/50 gas and air mixture (Entonox) self-administered by women in labour. In this case, a trained dentist administers and adjusts the mixture to get the optimum painkilling effect.

- An **intravenous anaesthetic** is an analgesic for very nervous patients. A dose of a Valium-type tranquillizer is injected into a vein in the forearm. Although patients can still feel pain and should have a local anaesthetic, they will not remember what happened. This form of anaesthesia is not suitable for the very young or old. There is a health risk, and all practices using this procedure must have two qualified people on the premises, and approved resuscitation equipment. Patients should not drive for some hours after receiving this, or relative anaesthesia.

- **Tranquillizers** are an alternative for nervous or phobic patients. They have the same effects as above but are taken prior to visiting the dentist in liquid or tablet form. You will need to visit your doctor for a prescription.

Temporary Dressings

These are used in emergencies, for example in a broken tooth or to treat a holiday toothache prior to proper treatment at your own dentist. Generally made of zinc oxide and eugenol (clove oil, which is bland and soothing to dentine) or glass-ionomer. However, even with added resins, zinc oxide is not robust and care must be taken when eating. Glass-ionomers are stronger. Dressings are also used when work is in progress on a tooth, such as with root treatments, temporary crowns, bridges and inlays.

Fillings

The dentist fills a tooth because it has become decayed, fractured or badly eroded. The decay, which is soft, has to be removed from the tooth in its entirety, using the drill and hand instruments. A cavity is cut to ensure that the filling stays in. Before either a white or amalgam filling is put in, a lining to protect the nerve is placed on the floor of the cavity. There are several types of filling (see Figure 10 below). These are:

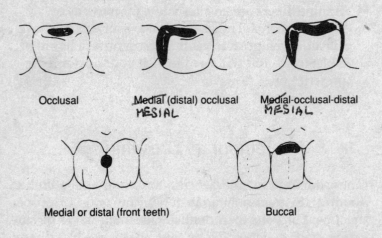

Occlusal

Medial (distal) occlusal
MESIAL

Medial-occlusal-distal
MESIAL

Medial or distal (front teeth)

Buccal

Figure 10 Types of filling

- Simple filling on the biting (*occlusal*) surface of a back tooth. (These are becoming rarer as the use of fluoride and sealing as preventive measures is taking effect.)
- Filling involving occusal surface and one or both of sides of the tooth between the teeth. The side nearer the middle is called *mesial*, the side further away is called *distal*. So you can have a mesial occlusal (MO), a distal occlusal (DO) or, if you are unlucky, a mesial occlusal distal (MOD).
- Sometimes the decay has spread to the inner surface (*palatal* at the top; *lingual* at the bottom) and/or outside walls (*buccal*) of the tooth. This may mean a filling will not be strong enough. Pins are sometimes inserted around which the filling is built – rather like piling for a building.
- The need for fillings on the front of the teeth near to the gum level can be caused by excessive wear from over-vigorous tooth brushing as well as by decay.
- Fillings between the front teeth. (These are becoming rarer with the use of fluoride.)
- Fillings to build up the corners of front teeth.

Amalgam fillings need to be packed firmly into the cavity cut by the dentist. The cavity is *'undercut'* (narrower at the top than the bottom). Amalgams are trimmed and polished. Composite fillings adhere to an acid-roughened tooth surface. The filling is built up layer by layer into a tooth shape, each layer being hardened by intensified light. It is very time-consuming. Glass-ionomers (which discharge fluoride) bond directly to the tooth, and are the easiest to use – unfortunately they are also the softest.

Sensitive Teeth

Sensitive teeth are caused by exposed dentine. This can be the result of shrinking gums, and heavy wear on the teeth (at the gum level or on the biting surfaces). In turn these can be caused by over-hard tooth-brushing, acids from the stomach, tooth grinding (*bruxism*), trauma or wear and tear. These can be self-treated by the avoidance of acid foods and the use of specialist toothpastes. However, if this does not work the dentist can fill the relevant areas or treat with fluoride paste.

Root Treatments

If either decay or trauma causes the nerve (pulp) of a tooth to die, a root treatment will be needed (see Figure 11).

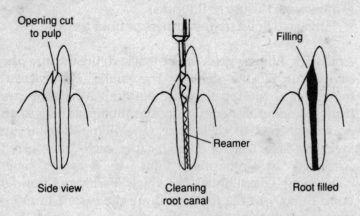

Figure 11 Root treatment

The pulp is removed with a thin hooked wire (*broach*), cleaned of infected and dead tissue, widened with reamers, and given a temporary filling of a sterile, thin column of compacted paper (*paper-point*), which may be impregnated with antibiotic or antiseptic solution. (If the infection is very acute, there may be an associated antibiotic course.) Only if there is no sign of infection at the next visit will the tooth be root-filled. Front teeth have a single root, 4s and 5s may have two roots, 6s and 7s tend to have three roots, but may have two or four, while 8s vary – upper 8s may have a single fused root. It is important to realize that in a root treatment all the root canals must be filled. In specialist *endodontic* surgeries, the equipment includes specialist microscopes, and electronic apex locators that detect the end of the root canal.

Apicectomies

These are surgical procedures that remove infected tissue around the tip of the root. They are done either when root treatments have failed or when they are not possible. They are performed under local anaesthetic by cutting into the gum and bone, drilling the infected bits of tooth and bone away, and filling the end quarter of the root canal with amalgam (*retro-filling*) before stitching (*suturing*).

Inlays

Inlays are cast fillings, cemented into the teeth. They may be gold, plastic or composite. They are used when an amalgam filling would be unsuitable, or when the tip of a front tooth is involved, or for personal aesthetic reasons. The dentist cuts the cavity in similar fashion as a filling. An impression is taken. Another impression is taken of the opposite jaw to show how the teeth interlock in the mouth (the *bite*). A dental laboratory technician makes the inlay, which the dentist cements into the tooth at the next visit, a 'temporary dressing' having been put into the cavity in the interim.

Crowns

Crowns, or 'caps' as they are also popularly known, are made for both front and back teeth (see Figure 12). They are used either when a tooth is no longer fillable conventionally or by inlay, or for aesthetic or cosmetic reasons. They are generally made of porcelain bonded onto a thimble of precious metal (often gold). There are three stages in the making of a crown. These are preparation, impression and fitting.

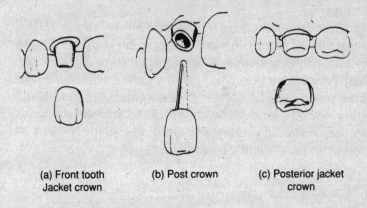

(a) Front tooth   (b) Post crown   (c) Posterior jacket
Jacket crown   crown

Figure 12

Preparation

The preparation is different for live and dead teeth. Live teeth are prepared by reducing the size of the tooth in all dimensions and preparing a good collar around the gum, against which the crown will fit. If the tooth is dead and root-filled, most of the tooth in the mouth is cut-away, leaving a collar as above. A post is made, or a pre-formed post is used for insertion into the root canal (in back teeth pre-formed posts are placed in all the root canals). This looks like a screw – hence the idea that these crowns are 'screw-in teeth'. The post(s) carry a stump of shaped filling material which has been built up to be a similar shape and size to the preparation on a live tooth.

Impression

Impressions are taken in the same way as for inlays, with two additions. An impression of the opposing teeth is taken, along with a sheet of wax showing how the teeth close together. This is so the crown will fit into the bite properly. The colour of the ceramic is also taken from a shade guide. The crown is made by a technician in the dental laboratory matching the shape as well as colour to the patient's own teeth.

Fitting

Between the preparation and the fitting of the crown, a temporary crown is put in position. The final crown is cemented onto the thimble, with care being taken to ensure that it fits precisely and meets the opposing teeth properly. Actors and politicians who are interested in their appearance often have all their crowns made on the same day in the same building.

Bridges

Bridges replace missing teeth. They are attached permanently to other teeth in the mouth. There are various types of bridges, carrying varying numbers of replacement teeth (*pontics*). The concept is the same in all of them, however. It is to use teeth (generally on either side of the gap) to support the replacement teeth. The supporting teeth act as the piers on a river bank supporting a bridge (see Figure 13).

There are four main forms of bridges: fixed/fixed, fixed/moveable, Maryland and cantilever.

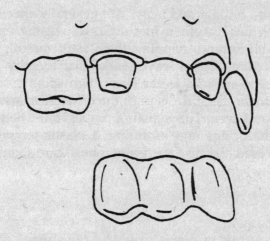

Figure 13 Bridge replacing one tooth

Fixed/fixed

Let us suppose that an upper 4 tooth (*first premolar*) has been lost. Crown preparations are made on the teeth either side of the gap – the upper 5 and the upper 3. Impressions are taken as for a crown. But instead of just making crowns the laboratory will make a metal framework on which three porcelain teeth, carefully colour-matched and shaped, are bonded. The centre tooth is a false one. The other two are supporting crowns on the upper 5 and upper 3. The whole is then cemented onto the upper 5 and upper 3 preparations. All vertical fitting surfaces must be parallel, otherwise the bridge cannot fit. The bridge must not press unduly on the teeth in the opposite jaw. It may need some time to be adjusted (*eased*) – as do all crowns and inlays. 'Easing' is self-explanatory. It is the removal of material from a crown, bridge, inlay or denture to make it comfortable.

For crowns, bridges and inlays this generally affects the way teeth bite together. In such cases, easing entails patients biting and grinding their teeth on coloured strips of paper. These leave marks that identify high spots on the artificial teeth. These high spots are then ground down using drills until the coloured marks are uniform and even. This signals a proper 'bite'. Between cutting the bridge and its fitting, a plastic temporary bridge is used. Because this is not robust, care should be exercised when eating.

Fixed/moveable

The idea of this bridge is to spread the stresses of the loads put on the bridge when biting or chewing. Too many bridges use teeth that are in no position to support a replacement tooth over long periods. One side of the bridge is made as before with a crown – let us say on the upper 5 (because it is likely to be the more stable). But the upper 3 crown (or inlay) is joined to the replacement tooth by a joint, which allows for some movement. This spreads the stresses, lessening the effects on both supporting teeth. In turn this increases the life of the bridge by increasing the life of the supporting teeth.

Maryland bridge

The Maryland technique is an example of minimal dentistry. The replacement tooth is attached to the teeth on either side of the gap with 'wings' of metal whose tooth-fitting surfaces have been specially prepared. The tooth surfaces of the adjacent teeth are acid-etched and composite filling material bonds the bridge to the enamel of both teeth. There can also be a hybrid, half-Maryland and half-conventional bridge.

Cantilever Bridge

The replacement tooth is suspended from one side only. The suspension can be of the Maryland type or a conventional crown. It is most often used to replace an upper 2, the replacement tooth being attached to the adjacent upper 3 only, leaving the upper 1 on the other side untouched.

Sticky (Adhesive) Dentistry

This is a newer set of techniques that uses various bonding substances for crowns, bridges, veneers, sealings and fillings. Traditional dentistry has been based on mechanical bonding using large cavities, and the removal of much tooth substance. Sticky dentistry, named after these new 'sticky' filling materials such as glass-ionomers, and the adhesives that join 'etched' tooth surfaces to artificial replacements of tooth substance, is much more tooth- and patient-friendly. It may well be the basis of most future restorative and replacement dentistry – other than dentures.

Implants

These are used to replace missing teeth. Metal posts are placed in the jawbone. Bone rejects most metals but under particular conditions, titanium has the property of *osteo-integration*. This means bone grows around, and can even cover, a titanium implant (see Figure 14). The two main conditions are (1) that the bone is prepared (drilled) very slowly, and (2) that the temperature is kept at a constant 4°C. There are several types of implant available, each requiring a slightly different technique.

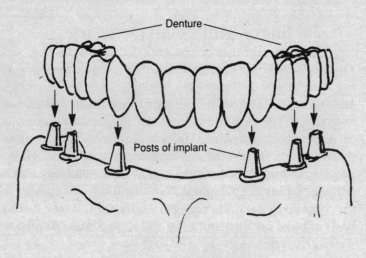

Figure 14 Titanium implant

The gum is opened to expose the bone. The hole is drilled. The titanium post is inserted, with about 1cm in the mouth. The gum is stitched. The post insertion may be done in two stages, the first stage being the insertion of a threaded sleeve, the second the screwing in of the post some two months later. The success rate is almost wholly dependent on proper planning and expertise. Specialist imaging – not just x-rays – is needed. The correct number of posts, their angles and load bearing need to be calculated beforehand. Once in, the implants can be used in two basic ways:

- As posts for one or more crowns or bridges. These are made in the same way as normal crowns and bridges and screwed onto the post. Patients are now starting to call these 'screw-in' teeth.
- As a basis for a denture. This is clipped onto the posts and, like all dentures, is removable.

Implants are extremely expensive. You will not get much change, if any, from £2000 for each unit. They must be made by highly experienced operators. They have a high degree of failure if proper care and planning are not exercised. A difficulty in this regard comes when an oral surgeon doing the implant and the conservationist or prosthetist making the superstructure do not communicate adequately at the planning stage.

Dentures

Dentures are probably the hardest thing to get completely right in the whole of dentistry. They can be partial (replacing some teeth) or full (replacing all the teeth). Most are made of acrylic (plastic) and have plastic, anatomically correct teeth. There are also skeleton partial dentures made of chrome-cobalt steel. These are made for patients unable to tolerate a full covering to the roof of the mouth, or for people who are allergic to acrylic plastics. They are expensive. Full upper dentures generally cover the roof of the mouth. Lower full dentures should cover as much of the floor of the mouth as possible. Both upper and lower partial dentures can be smaller, especially if the remaining teeth have metal clasps acting as anchors. There are also 'immediate dentures' (see Chapter 9, page 83). The four main stages in making a denture are: the impressions, the bite, the try-in and the fitting.

The impressions
These are taken in '*trays*' (see Chapter 11, page 101) with alginate-based impression material, from which plaster casts are made by the technician.

The bite
This is most important. It measures both the vertical height at which your teeth should meet when the mouth is comfortable, and the horizontal relationship between the upper and lower jaws. It is done by using carved pink wax slabs known as '*bite blocks*'. Tooth colour is selected at this stage.

The try-in
The technician has made the body of the denture(s) in wax, but with the final teeth. They are tried in the mouth to ensure the '*bite*' is correct, they look good and that the teeth mesh together *(articulate)* correctly. The

technician is given the correct try-in, and makes it in acrylic.

The fitting

It is unusual for a denture to be perfect at the fitting stage. It may well need a little easing, both on the pink acrylic where it rests on the gums, palate and the part of the gums that merge with the cheeks or floor of the mouth (*sulcuses*), and the teeth. If there is any pain, soreness or ulceration in these areas, or a denture supporting or opposing tooth starts to hurt, you should return to the dentist for an 'easing'. Part of this process is the same as for crowns, inlays and bridges (see above). However, a denture may also need easing on its fitting surface where it is in contact with the gums. It is often possible to see the parts that need easing from excessive redness, or perhaps a small ulcer. The easing is done by smoothing or removing small parts of the denture until it feels comfortable.

Gum Disease Treatments

The main objective in treating gum disease (*periodontal disease*) has changed from surgical intervention to plaque and calculus removal and managing a patient's oral hygiene. This starts with a *'periodontal charting'* (technically called the CPTIN) and detailed instructions in oral hygiene, tooth brushing, flossing, etc. The chart is used to compare the pocketing after 6 weeks then at intervals of 3 months. If the oral hygiene has improved and, as a consequence, pocket depth has decreased, the outlook for saving the teeth is good, providing the pockets were not too deep in the first place. Gum treatment is based on scalings, improved oral hygiene, and – in later stages – surgical intervention.

Scalings

Scalings are done by a dentist or a dental hygienist, using either ultrasonic or hand scalers, or both. Removal of gross *calculus* from the teeth in the mouth is straightforward, if time-consuming. Removing calculus entirely from beneath the level of the gums is a delicate matter. It can be uncomfortable, especially if there is exposed dentine on some of the teeth. To do this when advanced gum disease is present can be slow (no more than four teeth in a session) and may require a local anaesthetic. It is, however, a vital procedure, and is worth the discomfort. Without removing this deep calculus, the chances of arresting pocket formation, and so saving the teeth, are very slim.

Root planing

In essence this is scaling the length of the root within a pocket to remove calculus.

Gingivectomy

This is an operation to improve access to the surface of the tooth by removing the wall of the pocket (i.e. part of the gum itself). It allows for proper cleaning. The area is 'packed' with a gauzy dressing until healed. Gingivoplasty, which involves recontouring the gums, is a similar operation. Neither operation is done as often as in the past, partly because they were less than totally successful, and partly because the treatment of choice is now the management of the patient's plaque.

Surgery

This involves cutting the gum above (or below) the tooth and peeling it back to expose the bone, and the side and root of the tooth (if there is a deep pocket). This is called a surgical flap. The area is then scaled and cleaned. The gum is sutured in a slightly different position, exposing more of the tooth and allowing better access to this area for cleaning. It is possible to use bone chips in an attempt to get bone regeneration and/or go on a local antibiotic regime by packing the pocket with antibiotic gel or cord.

Splints

This treatment involves the use of a healthy tooth to stabilize an unstable one. It uses the same principle as strapping two fingers together to protect a broken one. This can be done with wires, Maryland technique or composite filling material.

Occlusal equilibration

This is intended to even up the biting pressure on teeth, so relieving the most vulnerable teeth, and/or stresses on the *tempero-mandibular joint* (TMJ), or jaw joint (see page 133 below). It is done by getting the patient to chew on pieces of coloured paper. These leave marks on the teeth where they strike first. The teeth are 'eased' in those places. The same technique is used to adjust inlays, crowns, bridges and dentures.

Root extraction

If the gums recede so far on some back teeth, naturally, or as a result of one of the above treatments, a root may be very exposed in the mouth. One root of a three-rooted tooth may need to be extracted – amputated would be a better description.

Extractions

Teeth are only extracted as a last resort, or as part of other treatment (see Orthodontics below). Extractions are normally done under local anaesthetic. Most extractions are straightforward and do not require brute strength; indeed all too many are of very loose teeth. They are performed with specialized forceps, which grip tightly on the crown of the tooth. The dentist expands the tooth socket, breaking the fibres holding the tooth to the bone by exerting steady pressure, and removes the tooth. On occasion, however, there may be difficulties. After extractions it is important to remember the following:

- Do *not* wash or spit out, eat or drink for several hours. Do not do heavy work or exercise for several hours. This is to allow a blood clot to form and healing to start.
- If bleeding re-starts, rest in a comfortable position

and bite hard on a rolled up handkerchief or kitchen towel for 20 to 30 minutes. Pressure stops bleeding. If the bleeding does not stop either return to your dentist or contact the emergency dental services.

- If, after one or two days, you get an intense, constant pain from where the tooth was extracted, which may also affect the teeth either side, you have a slightly infected socket (known as 'dry socket'). Although painful it is not serious. Return to your dentist who will treat it.

Surgical Extractions and Impacted Wisdom Teeth

These extractions are performed if a normal extraction technique fails (if the tooth breaks, for example) or of impacted teeth. They involve cutting the gum, removing bone to get access to tooth, pieces of tooth or root, removing them and suturing. They are generally performed under local anaesthetic, although severely impacted lower wisdom teeth may require a general anaesthetic. Wisdom teeth problems were covered in Chapter 8 (pages 69–70).

Orthodontics

This is an entire speciality of dentistry devoted to straightening malaligned teeth, and improving a person's dental and facial appearance. There are two major forms of malalignment. In one form the jaw relationship is abnormal and in the other the teeth are malaligned (crooked). Orthodontics deals with them both, and the two forms can be exhibited in one person. There are two main abnormalities of jaw relationship. Teeth are supposed to close with the front upper teeth just in front of, and in contact with and overlapping the bottom ones. In what is referred to as a Class II abnormality, a so-called 'weak-chin', the upper teeth protrude too much. A more prominent lower jaw with the lower teeth biting in front of the upper ones is called Class III. This may be the more difficult to treat successfully. Crowded teeth, overlapping teeth, crooked teeth, missing teeth and gaps between teeth are also dealt with. When these are found in a 'normal' biting position it is called Class I.

Orthodontic treatment is based on the fact that continuous, light pressure applied to a tooth can move it in the bone, and that the bone itself can be expanded or encouraged to grow – in other words develop to its own genetic potential. Most orthodontic treatment is carried out in the age bracket that spans the start and end of puberty. It can, however, start at ages as young as 5, and there is no upper age limit at all. Indeed, adult treatment is becoming ever more popular. The basic forms of orthodontic treatment are built around various forms of appliances, including the following.

- **Functional appliances** are removable appliances designed to improve or release the growth potential of the jaws. Examples include appliances with screws that expand the plate to widen the roof of the mouth (*palate*), or others that counteract muscular forces that may be stopping the lower jaw from growing. Functional appliances are used where there are skeletal difficulties, and they precede other treatments. Should treatment be carried out at very young ages it will almost certainly be with this form of appliance.

- **Fixed appliances** are bonded to the teeth. Typically they look like the miniature railway track seen on so many teenagers. Wires apply pressure to individual teeth to move them into the desired position. A typical treatment time is 21 months. However to stop the teeth 'relapsing' into their previous positions a minimum period of 1 year of stabilization with a moveable appliance is required. However, this stabilization might require more time, perhaps until the end of the normal growth period (17 or 18 years of age).
- **Removable appliances** are most often a plastic plate with wires and/or springs or screws that apply pressure to selected teeth, to move teeth relative to other teeth. This type of appliance is now more often used to maintain changed relationships, rather then changing the relationship in the first instance.

It may be that space has to be made to straighten the teeth, so one or more teeth have to be extracted, often, but not always, before an appliance is made and fitted.

The most noticeable functional appliance is one attached to a large metal bow sticking out from either side of the head. It looks like an extra-large pair of electrodes for Frankenstein's monster. It is capable of exerting large forces on the teeth.

Occasionally jaw surgery is needed, in addition to 'normal' orthodontic treatment, to correct misplaced teeth and jaw discrepancies.

Given patient cooperation and expert treatment

planning, there is every reason to believe that nearly 100 per cent of orthodontic treatments will succeed.

Transplanting a Knocked-out Tooth

This is the replacement of a permanent tooth (normally a front one) after it has been knocked out intact, most often as the result of an accident. The tooth should be kept moist with saliva in the cheek (or in milk). Do not try to clean it at all, leave bits of tissue or blood attached to it. Try to get to the dentist very quickly – do not phone for an appointment. The dentist will replace the tooth in the socket and splint it with adjacent teeth if possible. If you can do these things the results of implantation are fair. But once the tooth has been cleaned with tap water or detergents, or if there is delay, the chances are bad. The tooth will need to be root-treated later.

Shields

One way of avoiding this form of sporting accident is to wear a gumshield. While this can be purchased 'off-the-peg', the best ones are tailor-made by your dentist as they fit snugly around your teeth and gums. The dentist does this by taking an impression and having the shield made in a soft plastic.

Bruxism and Bite Raisers

Everyone grinds their teeth at night, if only a little. However, some people do it to excess. Although small children can be very noisy, it does no damage to them. But in adults, bruxism can cause tooth loss on the biting surfaces, sensitivity and fracture. Wearing a soft plastic bite-guard (*bite-raiser*) at night can minimize the damage.

Jaw Joint (TMJ)

The tempero-mandibular joint, or TMJ for short, is the hinged joint that enables the lower jaw to move. There are conditions, such as arthritis or a slipping disc, that make it painful to open wide, even to eat. One of the first stages of treatment may be to wear a *bite-raiser*. However, it may require surgery to correct the condition.

Cosmetic Dentistry

Cosmetic dentistry is dentistry done exclusively to improve or change a patient's appearance. It can be carried out by any dentist, although NHS options are limited. It includes replacing malformed, misplaced, or permanently discoloured teeth, as well as satisfying those who are searching for the perfect row of white teeth. Most cosmetic dentistry is concerned with crowns and bridges, although veneers are playing an increasingly important role. Some people like to adorn their teeth in a distinctly non-toothlike manner. While the Aztecs used to inlay emeralds, diamonds and rubies into their front teeth, gold is now the preferred cosmetic. Gold inlays, crowns and veneers (which have the advantage of not needing to cut into a healthy tooth as they are bonded onto the tooth) are being made in increasing numbers. Patterns in gold are also popular. Bleaching is another cosmetic treatment, but at the time of writing it is banned by the European Union, because of confusion about whether it is a cosmetic or pharmaceutical product. However, after a similar confusion it is now available in the USA. It lightens tooth colour very efficiently.

Lumps and Bumps

Aphthous ulcers are common in the mouth. They occur on the soft tissue over bone, in other words at the top and bottom of the gums. They are often associated with stress or the early stages of viral infections, but no-one knows exactly what causes them. Herpes ulcers or 'cold sores' on the lips also affect a significant percentage of people. There are many bumps in the mouth, some associated with the salivary glands: the *parotids* (in the cheek) and the *submandibulars* (under the tongue). Others are associated with the tongue, lips and cheek. Matching bumps on either side of the mouth or tongue are almost certainly natural, and indeed the great majority of lumps and bumps are *benign*. That is to say they are not cancerous (*malignant*). However, cancers do occur in the mouth, at roughly the same rate of incidence as malignant melanomas (runaway moles) or cervical cancers, and they have similar survival rates. 'Rodent ulcers', which are associated with sunlight, can be found (among other parts of the face) on the lips. They spread only locally and can easily be treated. Other cancers, however, called *squamous cell carcinomas*, can create more problems by spreading more widely and quickly. The earlier these cancers are detected and treated, the better the chance of complete cure. The difficulty, however, is that they can take many different forms. They may appear as ulcers, red lesions, white lesions or even wart-like lumps. By and large, they will be found on the side of the tongue, the floor of the mouth or the lower gums. And in the early stages, pain is no guide. They may be painless, give mild discomfort or considerable pain. So early diagnosis is difficult. But it is better to be safe than sorry. Any ulcers or bumps that last for more than two weeks, and are on the tongue, lips or cheeks, should take you to the dentist. If they cannot be explained by a denture fault, rough tooth or filling it is likely that you will be sent for a small sample to be checked by a pathologist *(biopsy)*, to find out what is wrong. It is extremely important that elderly people, especially those who wear full dentures and are accustomed to the odd sore patch or pain, take notice of this two-week warning.

Full Mouth Rehabilitation

This is, perhaps, a fancy name for a complicated set of treatments (when orthodontic treatment is inappropriate) for people whose teeth do not bite together properly. In turn this gives rise to a series of problems, including generalized pain, loose teeth, gum disease, excessive wear on some teeth, and TMJ problems. The treatment, which is designed to improve the articulation (biting position) of the teeth, involves extensive crown and bridge work, surgical procedures and implants. Most often it also involves considerable time and expense.

Chapter Fourteen

A Glimpse of the Future Today: Changes in Dentistry

Dental technology is changing. New ideas, equipment and materials, many based on new technologies, fill the specialist dental magazines. While many of them are still in the development stage, it is worth outlining some of the equipment you may see in private practice or in a dental hospital. Most will not be available in NHS general practice for some time, if ever.

Materials

New filling materials, however, will be universally available. Tooth-coloured filling materials with similar properties as the substance of a tooth will not be long delayed, probably developed from the line of products that have evolved from the nose tiles of space shuttles. They will be based on the 'sticky dentistry' principle. This will enable amalgam to be phased out. But initially they will be expensive. This is a fundamental point in the development of dental equipment and materials. In business generally, costs and prices fall with increasing volumes of sales. But dentistry is a limited market, so the more expensive equipment will almost certainly remain expensive, and out of the reach of NHS dentistry as it is currently constituted.

Computers

Personal computers are the classic example of increasing volumes of sales reducing prices, almost while you watch. Many dentists already chart on a computer, and some are on-line to the NHS authorities. But computers may well have another, more direct use. Computer-aided design and manufacture (CAD-CAM) is a well-established industrial process in which engineering design and manufacturing phases are merged using computers. Experiments with such a system, modified to allow a dentist to make ceramic crowns in the surgery as he or she works on the tooth, are now well under way, with more than a little success. An EU-funded study is experimenting with the uses of 'virtual reality' in this area of dentistry. This would enable a dentist to work on a tooth – but away from the patient – with a tiny robot clamped to the tooth, actually doing the physical work.

Lasers

Lasers are being used in a very limited number of private practice dental surgeries. As they can be focused and manipulated to different strengths, they are being used to 'dissolve' decay and seal teeth. In theory they could also be used in root canal treatments and gum surgery. Vibrationless, and painless (even in the absence of anaesthetics), they would represent a radical breakthrough if their capital and running costs were not prohibitively high. In an experiment in Tayside, ten dentists are using a new water-absorbing laser (the teeth do not heat up), but the equipment costs £40,000.

Implant Techniques

Implants cannot be performed on the NHS, mainly because the public purse will not meet the expense, even in part, but also because so few dentists are qualified to visualize, plan, make and fit them. However, one additional problem has been a lack of appropriate visualizing techniques – ordinary x-rays are not acceptable. This argues that ultrasound and *magnetic resonance imaging* (MRI) might find a place in 'dental implant centres', which are surely not that many years away. In the meantime the pan-oral x-ray machine, which provides a flattened full mouth x-ray picture, is used in implants, along with other x-rays taken at non-traditional angles.

X-rays

Pan-oral x-rays have been used in hospitals for many years, and indeed are used extensively in orthodontic departments. While some general dental practices are starting to use them, a simpler version is to add an attachment to standard practice modern x-ray machines which virtually turns them into wide-angle cameras. When the pictures are tacked together a pan-oral x-ray is obtained. A further advance in imaging technology is real-time imaging. Although it looks like, and is interpreted like, an x-ray, in fact it is another computer technique.

The Changing Face of Dental Practice

Dental practice itself is also likely to change. While this is partly because government clearly is unwilling to foot the NHS bill, the main reason is that dental expectations are rising. The only way they can be met, at a cost that the majority of people can meet, is to change the basis of dental practice. Routine dentistry may see a greater role for dental ancillaries – a sort of periodontal service. Dentists would then be able to concentrate on diagnosis, treatment planning and the more complex procedures.

Two things must be in place before this can happen. Increased facilities for training dental ancillaries and increased facilities for the training of dentists in specialities like implant technique and crown and bridge work. The General Dental Council, the body that controls the standards and ethics of dentists, is shortly to start along this road by maintaining registers of 'specialists', all of whom will have undergone appropriate training, and acquired appropriate qualifications. For the cost advantages to come through, such specialities could be provided in specialist centres, or at the very least dentists should work through a bulk-ordering cooperative for equipment and materials. The alternative will see a widening gap between dental expectations and the delivery of healthy mouths. But it has to be recognized that it is highly unlikely that any government will be able to fund the demand for more complex procedures such as implants.

Prevention and Toothpastes

A chemical and anti-bacterial approach to tooth and gum problems has been worked upon for many years. Inoculation against decay was the favoured option, but trials have always been disappointing. Suddenly, however, this line of anti-bacterial research appears to be bearing fruit. Indeed, new announcements and products are appearing in quick succession, almost on a monthly basis.

A good example is a very new product, developed in late 1995 in association with the Royal London Dental Hospital, appears to have the property of preventing, halting and even reversing dental decay. It is a varnish, which when applied by dentists to root decay (see Chapter 9) at 3 monthly intervals, actually produced new calcification in over half the cases. This means it not only stopped the decay, it protected the area against further attacks by acids and bacteria. Its ingredients work by reducing the number of decay-producing bacteria on the tooth. Clearly this has vast potential in curing decay as well as prevention. It also has the virtue of relative cheapness.

A whole new range of readily available mainstream toothpastes which now use oxidisation agents as well as fluoride, works in a similar way. Look for pastes labelled with 'anti-bacterial system' or an ingredient such as 'tricosan'. A newer toothpaste, not yet in the high street shops, uses substances which virtually 'tranquillize' these bacteria. This product is also available as a spray, and early research backs up the claims that it acts on gum disease bacteria too, as well as whitening teeth and freshening breath. If this early promise proves to be justified, this anti-bacterial approach might herald the beginning of a very different form of dentistry, better dental self-help, and the end of decay for most people's teeth.

Chapter Fifteen

Alternative Dentistry

Alternative medicine has captured both the imagination and the allegiance of a substantial minority of people, for part or indeed all of the time. While an osteopath could be consulted about trouble with the jaw joint, the main branches of alternative medicine that might be used in dentistry are more likely to be hypnosis, acupuncture, herbalism and homeopathy.

Combating Fear

Many people are scared of the dentist, others are scared of dental surgeries, and yet others are scared of both. While most people can cope, at the worst this is a fully-fledged phobia. It is possible to use tranquillizers of various descriptions, and certainly to receive the relative anaesthesia we outlined earlier. There are also various relaxation techniques, tapes and videos available. But some people just cannot get to the dentist at all, while others get there only to freeze into terrified immobility. For such people, hypnosis may be the only answer. The British Society of Medical and Dental Hypnosis trains doctors and dentists in hypnosis techniques, and will provide lists of their qualified practitioners practising in your area. The Society is regionally based, and their telephone numbers and addresses can be found in your local *Yellow Pages* – generally under 'Hypnotherapy'.

Homeopathic treatment can also be effective in dealing with the fears associated with visiting the dentist. Aconite, Argentum Nitricum and Gelsemium are homeopathic remedies that have all been tried with some success. However, it is important to realize that homeopathy treats the individual rather than the complaint. In turn this means that what may work for one person may not work for another, so if you are serious in wanting to try homeopathy, consult a qualified homeopath who will match the remedy to you.

Homeopathic Treatment

Some homeopathic remedies are becoming part and parcel of everyday life, not to say conventional medicine. Arnica is used widely as a remedy for bruises, sprains and trauma, and is as much a part of the average medicine cabinet as TCP or Calpol. Arnica can be taken one day before and one day after dental treatment in order to minimize the effects of trauma, especially if extractions are expected. Other remedies include hypericum, which is specifically aimed at nerve damage (used after root treatments), and calendula, which treats bleeding from damaged tissues. These are combined in a tincture that may be diluted as a mouthwash (Hypercal). Mercurius can also be used as a remedy for spongy gums and excessive salivation. Indeed, almost all dental diseases or symptoms have a specific homeopathic remedy, all of which are detailed in the 'Teeth and Gums' section of *The Family Guide to Homoeopathy: The Safe Form of Medicine for the Future*, by Dr Andrew Lockie, Elm Tree Books, 1989.

Most remedies should be taken in either the 6c or 30c potency, and almost all can be found in tablet form. Although many mainstream pharmacies now stock homeopathic remedies, alongside dedicated homeo- pathic pharmacies, if you wish to try these remedies for dental purposes and are worried about the strength and frequency of the dosage, contact a professional homeopath. The Society of Homeopaths keeps a register of professionally qualified practitioners and the Faculty of Homeopathy has a list of medical doctors who also practise homeopathy. *Yellow Pages* is useful for finding addresses and telephone numbers, although personal recommendation is useful. There are also a number of dentists who are starting to engage with homeopathic remedies. You should ask around. One dental side effect of using any homeopathic remedy, for whatever reason, is that you should not use any mint-flavoured toothpaste or one with a fluoride additive.

Herbalism

Most 'alternative dentistry' cures for decay or the causes of abscesses and gum disease may be effective for symptoms, but may not be as effective at removing the underlying causes. In terms of symptoms, many herbal anti-inflammatory and painkilling compounds are available, and may be effective. They can, of course be used to ease some side effects of treatment as well. Nevertheless, Chinese herbalists claim to be able to cure gum disease or bad breath, both of which are related to the stomach in Chinese physiology, and given the impressive record of Chinese treatments it would be unwise to totally discount them. Equally, in dentistry it would be unwise to rely on them totally. Longer term you will still have to visit the dentist to have the cause of your discomfort or pain treated, whether it is due to decay or loss of bone around the teeth. There are several books on the subject of herbal remedies. An example is *Essential Book of Herbal Medicine*, by Simon Mills. If you are interested in this area you should visit either a herbal chemist or one of the growing number of herbal healers.

Acupuncture

If Chinese and other herbal remedies are used to treat the disease itself, acupuncture is used to treat its manifestations. This means it is used to relieve toothache, whether this is caused by decay or gum disease. However a visit to the dentist will still be necessary to deal with the underlying causes. Acupuncture relates the teeth to 'kidney essence function' and believes that a tendency to bad teeth is an inherited aspect. Acupuncture anaesthesia is also being used, and a small but increasing number of dentists are aware of it. The point of insertion is between the thumb and first finger, and the anaesthesia – which completely numbs all the teeth and gums – can be made to last for one hour. A visit or phone call to your local acupuncture clinic (they can be found in *Yellow Pages*) will give you all the information you need. However, acupuncture anaesthesia will require close cooperation between your dentist and an acupuncturist.

Glossary of Terms

This is a short selection of words and abbreviations that you might come across at the dental surgery, either in comments addressed to you or in overheard instructions or conversations between the dentist and the dental nurse. It is not intended to be an exhaustive dictionary, merely a guide to help you understand what is going on.

abrasion
Loss of enamel caused by physical non-tooth contact (often excessive tooth brushing).

abscess
Caused by white blood cells tackling a localized infection. May be acute (gumboil) or chronic (sinus draining into mouth).

acrylic
Plastic base of most dentures.

air-rotor
High-speed drill.

alginate
Impression material used in denture making, made from a substance extracted from seaweed.

amalgam
Filling material made from a mixture of mercury, copper, silver and zinc.

apex
The tip of the root of a tooth.

apical abscess
Abscess in the bone at the root tip. Most often results from a dead tooth.

apicectomy
Operation to remove infection at the tip of the tooth root (apex).

aphthous ulcer
Painful gum ulcer of unknown cause, more common in young people.

area
Patch of chronic infection at apex of tooth.

attrition
Wearing of teeth caused by other teeth (see **bruxism** below).

autoclave
Efficient sterilizer.

bite-wings
Type of x-ray to find bone loss and decay between teeth.

block
Injection at back of lower jaw, numbing all the lower side.

broach
Instrument used to remove pulp in root treatment procedures.

bruxism
Grinding of teeth – especially in sleep.

buccal
Side of tooth next to cheeks.

burr
The cutting part of a drill. Made of industrial diamond, steel or tungsten steel.

calculus
Calcified plaque laid down on teeth in the mouth and beneath the gums. Also deposited on dentures. Used to be known as tartar.

canine
Pointed tooth third from the mid-line. Also known as 'dog-tooth'.

caries
Tooth decay. Note also the adjective 'carious', meaning decayed.

Cavitron
Trade name of an ultrasonic scaler.

cavity
A grossly decayed part of the tooth or a hole cut by the dentist.

cement
Used to attach crowns, bridges, etc., to teeth.

cementum
Hard substance covering dentine on the root of a tooth.

charting
'Map' made by dentist of the number and position of teeth, existing dental work and work to be done.

chlorhexidine
Chemical that has the property of preventing the build-up of plaque.

chrome-cobalt steel
Metal used to make 'skeleton dentures'.

clasps
Metal hooks on teeth for dentures or orthodontic appliances.

Class I
Orthdontic description of normally aligned jaws, where the upper front teeth close in front of the lower front teeth.

Class II
Orthodontic condition where upper teeth protrude.

Class III
Orthodontic condition where lower jaw protrudes.

CPITN
Index of severity of gum disease used in charting.

dentine
The major part of the tooth, covered by enamel in the mouth and cementum on the root. It is sensitive.

diastema
Gap between teeth.

distal
The side of the tooth away from the centre of the mouth.

DO
Two-surface filling in back teeth: back and biting surface.

dressing
Temporary filling.

elevator
Instrument used in helping to extract teeth or roots.

enamel
Hard, insensitive outer covering of the tooth crown (in the mouth).

erosion
Loss of enamel due to acid, age or tooth grinding.

excavator
Small, spoon-like instruments used to remove the last vestiges of decay from a tooth.

flanges
Part of dentures that extend down into the base of the cheek.

fluorosis
Mottling of enamel caused by excess intake of fluoride.

frenum
Centrally placed tissue strand connecting the inside of the top lip to the gum.

gingival pocket
Gap between gum and tooth caused by deposition of plaque and calculus.

gingivitis
Inflammation of the gums – start of gum disease.

glass-ionomer
White filling material that adheres to dentine and releases fluoride. Suitable for non-biting surface fillings.

hygienist
Person who scales teeth and gives oral hygiene instruction.

impacted
Teeth unable to erupt properly, such as wisdom teeth.

incisor
Spade-shaped front tooth. There are eight incisors.

inlay
Cast filling.

lignocaine
Most commonly used local anaesthetic.

lingual
The side of a lower tooth next to the floor of the mouth.

lining
Barrier put between a filling and floor of cavity.

Maryland
A type of adhesive bridge.

mesial
The side of the tooth towards the centre of the mouth.

MO
Two-surface filling in back teeth: front and biting surface.

MOD
Three-surface filling in back teeth.

mucocele
Small, harmless but irritating lump, commonly on lips.

mucosa
Lining of mouth, cheeks, gums, etc.

occlusal
Biting surface of back teeth; also filling on this surface.

palatal
The side of an upper tooth next to the roof of the mouth.

pan-oral
Type of full-mouth x-ray.

parotid
Salivary gland situated in the cheek.

pericoronitis
Inflammation around the crown of a wisdom tooth.

periodontal
Around the tooth, as in 'periodontal abscess'.

periodontitis
Advanced gum disease, formerly known as pyorrhea.

pocketing
See **gingival pocket**.

pontic
The replacement (not supporting) element of a bridge.

probe
Small, pointed, right-angled hand instrument used in charting and checking.

pulp
Soft tissue running down the centre of the root(s) containing the blood and nerve supply of a tooth.

pyogenic granuloma
Excessive localized growth of gum tissue, often associated with pregnancy.

ridges
Bony part of mouth on which dentures sit.

sinus
Drainage channel connecting chronic abscess to mouth.

squamous cell carcinoma
Most common form (90 per cent) of internal mouth cancer.

sticky dentistry
Term referring to crowns, bridges, etc., cemented onto or into teeth.

submandibular
Salivary glands situated in floor of mouth.

sulcus
Space between the gum and cheeks.

tartar
Old name for **calculus.**

TMJ
Tempero-mandibular joint where lower jaw hinges onto upper jaw.

Index

Index

Let's Eat Right to Keep Fit

Adelle Davis

Here Adelle Davis presents information concerning our bodies' vital nutritional processes which is both authoritative and fascinating. Her recommendations for a balanced diet are important for anyone interested in preventive medicine.

Over 40 nutrients needed by the body for health are discussed in detail and the foods that supply them are listed.

Described by *Time* magazine as 'the highest authority in the kitchen', the value of good wholesome food over synthetic foods is stressed throughout. This book remains a bible for anyone interested in health or food – from doctors to cooks.

LET'S EAT RIGHT TO KEEP FIT   0 7225 3203 2   £5.99   ☐

This book is available from your local bookseller or can be ordered
direct from the publishers.

To order direct just tick the title you want and fill in the form below:

Name:

Address:

Postcode:

Send to Thorsons Mail Order, Dept 3, HarperCollins*Publishers*,
Westerhill Road, Bishopbriggs, Glasgow G64 2QT.
Please enclose a cheque or postal order or your authority to debit
your Visa/Access account —

Credit card no:

Expiry date:

Signature:

— up to the value of the cover price plus:
UK & BFPO: Add £1.00 for the first book and 25p for each
additional book ordered.
Overseas orders including Eire: Please add £2.95 service
charge. Books will be sent by surface mail but quotes for airmail
dispatches will be given on request.

**24-HOUR TELEPHONE ORDERING SERVICE FOR
ACCESS/VISA CARDHOLDERS — TEL: 0141 772 2281.**